Deep Learning and Machine Learning Frameworks for Cervical Cancer Screening

treven
Shylok

TABLE OF CONTENTS

CHAPTER - 1: INTRODUCTION

1.1. CANCER

Worldwide, cancer is the primary cause of death, placing a heavy strain on those who are afflicted, their families, and the healthcare system. Five to ten percent of cancer cases are inherited. It is typified by unchecked cell proliferation brought on by a range of factors that can cause cancer either separately or in combination, including smoking, pathogenic organisms, somatic and germ line mutations, poor food, and internal factors. A certain bodily location started to develop abnormally as cancer started to emerge in the cells. Cancer can take many different forms, but all of them start when strange cells start growing abnormally. The capacity of a cancer cell to go wild and attack different tissues is what makes it unique. Metastasis is the word used to describe the spread of cancer cells to other parts of the body. These illnesses cover a wide spectrum of conditions where normal cells develop abnormally and affect any portion of the body. Cancers are categorized into squamous cell and epithelial cell subtypes based on their cellular origin. Certain cell types are the source of some cancers.

1.2. CERVICAL CANCER

The cervix uteri, the lowest point of the womb's neck in the female reproductive system, is the source of cervical cancer, a hazardous tumor that develops from those cells. The cervix is surrounded by glandular and squamous cells. Cervical malignancies that start in the uterus, at the vaginal junction, and in the core layer of the cervix are frequently caused by the human papillomavirus (HPV). It starts as dysplasis, a precancerous condition, and progresses slowly. Cancer is the top 10 causes of fatality in India, with an estimated 2-2.5 million humans affected by the disease (Sunget al., 2021). Most people agree that one of the most dangerous malignancies on the earth is cervical cancer.

The increased incidence of cancer identification at later stages among women in developing countries is associated with a worse prognosis and a higher death rate. This is probably because there are fewer therapeutic choices available. High-risk human papillomaviruses (HPV) are responsible for most cases of cervical cancer. human papillomaviruse is a highly contagious virus, accounting for 99 percent of cases. This type of cancer most commonly affects females between the ages of 14 and 45. Every year, cervical cancer claims the lives of about 200,000 women; in developing nations, almost 90% of deaths are related to a lack of access to healthcare and medical knowledge. Over 80% of instances of cervical cancer occur in underdeveloped nations, making it the most general cancer in many parts of the world. In recent decades, the broad implementation of cytologic screening programs has shown to be a methodical strategy for reducing cervical cancer's incidence and death rates.

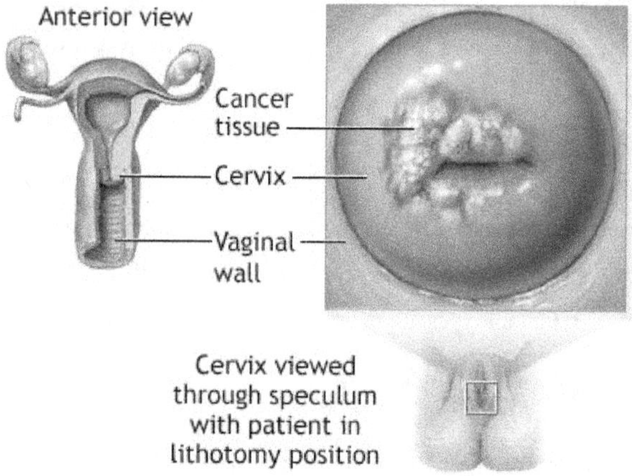

Figure 1.1 Cervical cancer

1.3. DIAGNOSTIC METHODS OF CERVICAL CANCER

The spread of cervical cancer is gradual and steady. Early changes can be detected with screening tests in conjunction with routine gynaecologic check-ups. If cervical cancer is discovered early on, it is completely treatable. To identify the underlying source of her problems, every woman needs to recognize these symptoms and seek medical guidance.

1.3.1. Types of Cervical Test

- **i.** Pap Smear test
- **ii.** HPV test
- **iii.** Colposcopy test

i. Pap smear Test

The physician takes a sample of cervical cells for the Pap smear test. It is used to split the cell over time and identify abnormal alterations in the cell's growth. Women between the ages of 21 and 29 are tested every three years. For women over 30, it takes place every five years. In addition to detecting cervical cell changes, the Pap smear test can detect infections that are not malignant. The number of fatalities from cervical cancer has significantly decreased since the Pap test was widely used. After receiving a Pap smear, many women choose not to return for follow-up tests or care. Many women diagnosed with cervical cancer never had a normal Pap test.

Papanicolaou (Pap smear) tests are the most effective means of preventing and detecting cancer. The steps in the traditional Pap test are as follows.

- The vagina is dilated to allow visualization of the cervix by inserting the speculum.
- Sample cells from inside and around the cervix are collected using brushes or swabs.
- To maintain cell viability in glass, a stabilizer is utilized.
- Samples are labelled to better reveal structural patterns for examination under a microscope in the lab by enhancing contrasts within the sample.

Normal V.S. Abnormal Cervical Cells

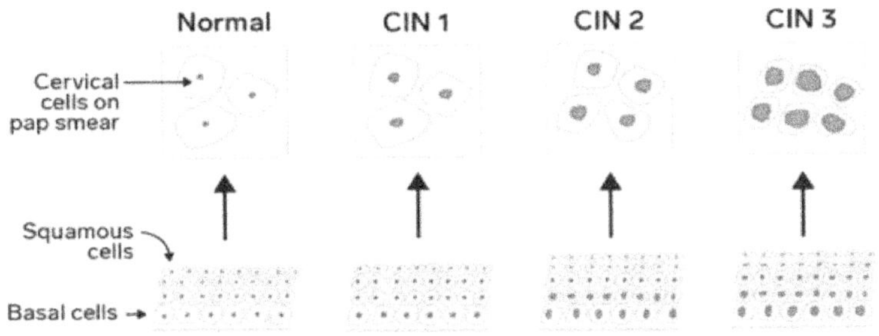

Figure 1.2 Pap Smear Samples Test Results

Limitations

The final report from a Pap smear test may take many days or weeks. Two important elements influence the Pap smear test's accuracy.

- First, an inadequate number of cervix samples are collected by a lab worker.
- Second, there was a misinterpretation by a lab professional.

Steps:

A sample of cells is obtained from the transformation zone for the Pap smear test is first taken using a brush or spatula. After that, this sample is spread out or put on a glass slide and fixed with a fixative to keep the cells from drying out. In order to improve contrast and enable the differentiation of tissues from background, the fixed sample is lastly coloured.

ii. HPV Test

The HPV test does not diagnose cancer; rather, it is used to screen for cervical cancer. Rather, the test searches for HPV, the virus that causes cervical cancer, within your system. To detect every piece of information pertaining to the condition, all of these tests have to be run simultaneously. It is recommended that these screening tests be conducted after the age of 21.

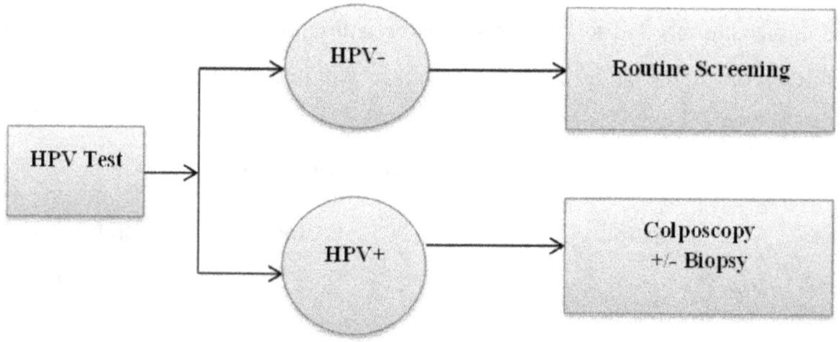

Figure 1.3 Pathway for HPV testing

iii. Colposcopy Test

Colposcopy is a method that involves closely examining your vulva, vagina, and cervix to look for signs of disease. A colposcopy is a specialized tool that your physician uses for the colposcopy procedure. Should the findings of your Pap test be abnormal, your physician can recommend a colposcopy. If your doctor detects an abnormal cell region during your colposcopy procedure, a sample of tissue may be removed for laboratory investigation (biopsy). Colposcopy procedures typically take ten to twenty minutes in a physician's office.

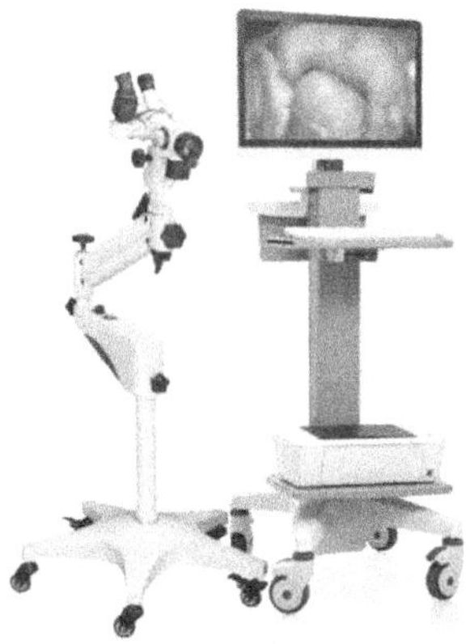

Figure 1.4 Device used for Colposcopy

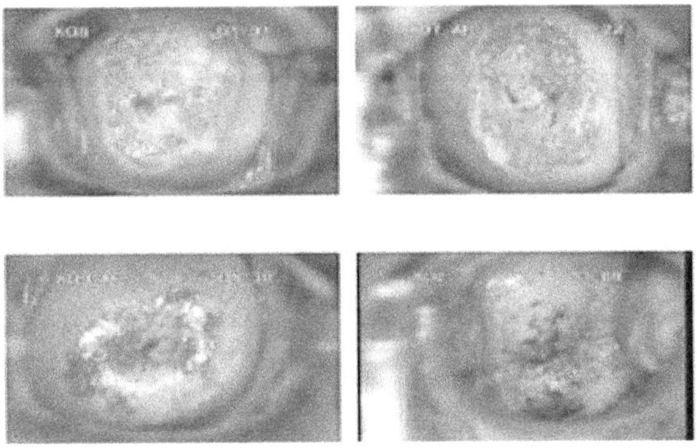

Figure 1.5 Colposcopy Cervical Cancer Image

1.3.2. Other Diagnostic Techniques

Imaging methods must be applied to the body to obtain an internal cervix image following a colposcopy. There are various image technique methods accessible, including:

- X-ray
- Computerized Tomography (CT) scan
- MRI stands for magnetic resonance imaging.

i) X-ray

X-rays and other electromagnetic waves are examples of radiation. X-ray imaging can be used to capture images of your inside organs. X-rays are used to identify soft tissue abnormalities, such as those affecting internal organs. X-ray technology is used to display 2D images.

ii) CT

Accurate information about an organ is provided by a CT scan, which is very beneficial for the therapeutic procedure. It provides intrinsic data on the organ in question and examines its blood channels and muscles. The patient experiences no pain during the CT scan process, and the results are obtained quickly. An organ's 3D pictures are displayed.

iii) MRI

MRI scans, as opposed to CT scans, which require high radiation levels, use a magnetic field to capture images. It can more successfully assist the practitioner in starting treatment by allowing them to visualize the precise structure of soft tissue organs. To take pictures, MRI imaging technology is used.

Stages of Cervical Cancer

Table 1.1 Various Stages of Cervical Cancer

Stage	Description	Stage types		Description
I	Cancer is generally detected in the cervix.	IA	IA1	The maximum depth of cancer is 3 mm, and the maximum width is 7 mm.
			IA2	The carcinoma is not deeper or wider than 7 or 5 mm, although it is larger than 3 mm.
		IB	IB1	Cancer 5 mm or more in deep and less than 2 cm
			IB2	Cancer is 2 cm or more in deep and smaller than 4 cm
			IB3	Cancer is at least 4 cm
II	Cancer will extend outside the cervix but not to the pelvic divider or the lowest portion of the vaginal canal.	IIA	IIA1	The tumor is 4 cm in diameter and visible without magnification.
			IIA2	There is no need for a microscope to see the tumour.
		IIB		Cancer will extend elsewhere the cervix to the tissues surrounding the uterus.
III	Cancer is spreading to the bottom vaginal area and the pelvic wall, causing kidney issues.	IIIA		The cancer has not yet penetrated the pelvic wall, However, it has extended to the vagina's lower region.
		IIIB		Only the pelvic wall has been impacted, not the lower part of the vagina.
IV	Cancer can also affect other organs, such as the rectum and bladder.	IVA		The bladder and rectum are among the adjacent organs where this cancer has progressed.
		IVB		Beyond the cervix, cancer will spread to other parts of the body.

1.4. PROBLEM STATEMENT

After a protracted infection, some stretches of the HPV can lead to cervical cancer. Sexually transmitted viruses, including the human papillomavirus (HPV), can cause these cancers. Although there are very few women who develop cervical cancer, at some point in their life, more than half of all sexually active people will get HPV. Most women diagnosed with cervical cancer today did not get screened at the recommended intervals. When a person is uncovered to HPV, their immune system usually stops the virus from doing any damage. Sixty-six percent of individuals with cervical cancer survived for five years. However, there are differences in survival rates based on age, race, and ethnicity. Although it usually advances slowly, cervical cancer can grow and spread quickly in some situations.

Most people agree that cervical cancer is curable with proper treatment, particularly if caught early. The cervix, or tube that joins the vagina and the bottom portion of the uterus, is impacted by this illness. The most common screening procedure for precancerous cells (dysplasia) and cervical cancer is the Pap test. Like many other tests, the Pap test has a key flaw in that it cannot ensure reliable results. The mixture of distorted images and cell pictures makes it challenging to divide the light in the microscope so that it is either overexposed or underexposed.

The fatality rates from cervical cancer have dropped because of the effectiveness of screening programs. However, cervical cancer screening remains a challenging process because most screening methods are invasive. This invasiveness often makes people hesitant to undergo standard screening procedures, and it also leads to longer waiting times for results.

The images produced by Papanicolaou (Pap) devices, while essential, come with certain limitations:

1. Issues in image acquisition can introduce noise, affecting the clarity of the results.
2. Variations in tissue thickness create contrasting areas, leading to irregularities in anatomical structures within the images.

1.5. OBJECTIVES

The following are the goals of the research methodologies:

1. Develop and implement an advanced deep learning model for cervical cancer diagnosis, using the latest techniques.
2. Integrate feature extraction techniques to enhance the diagnostic accuracy of the model for detecting various stages of cervical cancer.
3. To evaluate the performance of the proposed method against the existing diagnostic methods and state-of-the-art deep learning models.

This research aims to develop a dependable, automated method for detecting cervical cancer in colposcopy images. Type 1 (normal), Type 2 (low-grade lesions), and Type 3 (high-grade lesions or malignant) are the three categories into which the system will divide the photos. Early detection and precise cervical cancer diagnosis will be made easier by this classification, which will lessen the subjectivity and unpredictability involved with manual interpretations.

Specific Goals:

1. **Data Collection and Pre-processing**: Gather a sizable data set of colposcopy images and enhance their quality for analysis by preprocessing them to guarantee consistency.
2. **Feature Extraction**: Use advanced methods, such as the Histogram of Oriented Gradients (HOG) and the Gray Level Co-occurrence Matrix (GLCM), to extract pertinent information from the colposcopy pictures.
3. **Hybrid Feature Fusion**: Create a hybrid feature fusion vector by combining the extracted features to increase classification accuracy.
4. **Model Development**: To classify the colposcopy images, create and train a variety of machine learning classifiers, such as more conventional models like Random Forest and more sophisticated models like Convolutional Neural Networks (CNNs).

5. **Performance Evaluation**: Assess the classifiers' performance using metrics such as sensitivity, specificity, recall, F1-score, accuracy, and precision to identify the top-performing model.
6. **Implementation and Validation**: Implement the best-performing model and validate its performance on an autonomous test set of colposcopy images to ensure its reliability and generalizability.

1.6. THESIS ORGANIZATION

The thesis is organized into nine chapters, as outlined below:

Chapter 1: This chapter introduces the impact and severity of cervical cancer in female patients, providing an overview of the disease and its diagnostic challenges. The chapter also outlines the objectives of the research, emphasizing the development of advanced diagnostic frameworks for cervical cancer detection.

Chapter 2: A detailed literature survey is presented, highlighting conventional methods for cervical cancer diagnosis and their limitations. This chapter also reviews recent advancements in image processing and machine learning techniques applied to medical imaging.

Chapter 3: This chapter elaborates on the proposed diagnostic system, including data preprocessing, feature extraction methods such as GLCM and HOG, and hybrid feature fusion. It provides a comprehensive description of the framework and its integration with machine learning classifiers.

Chapter 4: The experimental results are discussed in this chapter, including performance evaluation metrics such as accuracy, precision, and recall. Comparative analyses of traditional and proposed methods are presented to validate the framework's efficacy.

Chapter 5: This chapter focuses on advanced machine learning models, particularly deep learning architectures, and their application to cervical cancer detection. It explores how convolutional neural networks (CNNs) and other modern techniques enhance classification performance.

Chapter 6: A detailed discussion of the fusion of traditional and modern feature extraction methods, along with an ensemble classification approach, is provided. The chapter highlights the synergy between these techniques in improving diagnostic outcomes.

Chapter 7: This chapter summarizes the development and evaluation of the ColpoClassifier framework. It emphasizes the significance of integrating image processing techniques with robust machine learning algorithms and provides insights into the experimental findings.

Chapter 8: This chapter presents additional analysis and validation of the framework, emphasizing the practical implications of the research findings for clinical applications and broader healthcare settings.

Chapter 9: The concluding chapter summarizes the key contributions of the research, reflecting on the significance of the proposed methodologies. It also discusses future research directions and the potential for further advancements in automated cervical cancer detection.

CHAPTER – 2: LITERATURE SURVEY

2.1. BACKGROUND

2.1.1. Image Processing

The Image processing is a method for enhancing or improving images and extracting the pertinent features. This type of processing involves signals. Picture processing is used in the medical sector to examine 3D picture files of the human body, usually obtained from an MRI or CT scanner. These files are utilized for research purposes, medical procedure guidance (e.g., surgery planning), diagnosis, and other purposes. Artificial Intelligence (AI) has been investigating all aspects of image processing in recent years. AI enables facial recognition and authentication, as well as the detection and identification of objects and patterns in pictures and videos. The two methods most frequently utilized for processing medical images are machine learning and deep learning.

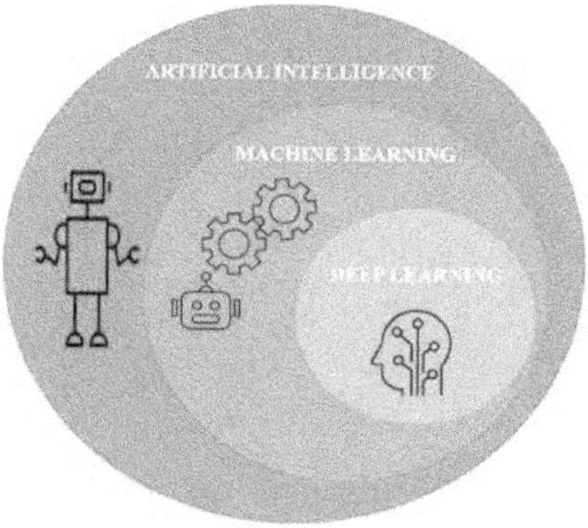

Figure 2.1 Types of AI

- **Machine Learning (ML)**

The ability of a machine to simulate intelligent human behavior is known as artificial intelligence. The science of automated systems that may improve over time by learning from data is known as machine learning (ML). Predictions are produced by an algorithm that builds a model using training data so that it can make decisions or predictions without having to be specifically programmed to do so. Three methods are used to do this: data processing, model construction, deployment, and monitoring.

Methods of Machine Learning

Four categories can be used to classify machine learning approaches:

- Data Science Supervised Machine Learning
- Data Analysis Using Unsupervised Machine Learning
- Machine Learning using Semi-Supervision
- Machine Learning Algorithms with Reinforcements

In **supervised ML**, Labelled examples allow them to apply their knowledge to new data and forecast future occurrences. The learning algorithm uses an analysis of a specific training dataset that I can build an inferred function for output value prediction with. After sufficient training is finished, the system will give goals for every new input. In order to allow for model correction, the learning algorithm can also identify errors by comparing its output with the desired one.

Unsupervised ML: An unsupervised learning strategy is applied when there is no classification or labelling in the training data. Computers can characterize hidden structures from unlabelled data using unsupervised learning. The system uses unlabelled datasets to find hidden structures rather than deciding what output to produce.

Semi-Supervised ML: This approach combines supervised and unsupervised learning. There is a little amount of marked data, and a huge number of unlabelled data used for training in semi-supervised learning. With this approach, learning accuracy in systems can be significantly increased. When training or learning from labelled data necessitates the utilization of qualified and sufficient resources, semi-supervised learning is popular. However, unlabelled data typically doesn't necessitate the utilization of extra resources.

Reinforcement ML Algorithms: In response to its surroundings, this algorithm determines successes and failures and produces actions accordingly. The features of reinforcement learning include delayed incentives and trial-and-error search. With the application of this technology, robots and software agents can become more productive by choosing their own behaviours based on the specifics of the circumstance. The agent needs a reinforcement signal—a straightforward reward—to figure out which action is optimal.

Here are a few instances of machine learning grouping algorithms in action:

- Naive Bayes Classifier
- K Nearest Neighbour
- Support Vector Machines
- Random Forest
- Boosted Trees
- Decision Trees
- AI Neural Network

Logistic regression is the simplest basic machine learning classifier; it uses a medical picture as a dependent variable and predicts its output. It is a probability value that falls between exact integers, such 0 and 1, such as Yes, No, 0, 1, true, false, and so on. It cannot accurately predict sickness based on a medical image. In order to address the issue, the Naive Bayes classifier was developed. It's an easy-to-use and efficient classification method that helps quickly develop machine learning models that can identify illnesses with less data in the image and generate accurate predictions. It is also accurate in class prediction. It functions better in comparison to logistic aggression. If a categorical variable that wasn't appears in the test set from the training set, Naive Bayes predict anything. It is not without restrictions, though. If a categorical variable that wasn't in the training set turns up in the test set, the Naive Bayes model won't be able to predict anything.

For more accurate illness identification in medical imaging After developing the K nearest neighbour classifier, it Predictions can be made without the requirement for training, and the accuracy of the image is unaffected by the addition of new data. KNN is a very effective tool, unable to operate with huge datasets. In order to address the shortcomings of k nearest neighbour, support vector machines (SVMs) were developed. SVMs are more efficient in high-dimensional areas. This approach performs effectively when there are more dimensions than samples. In order to get over SVM's drawbacks, like as noise and data set overlaps, underperform if there are more features per data point than there are training data samples. A decision tree is suggested; it shortens the training period and enables the system to process both categorical and continuous inputs. This classifier's flaw is over fitting of the data, which produces inaccurate predictions and is affected by noise in addition to failing to account for missing values.

To mitigate the drawbacks of the tree technique, Random Forest (RFC) was created. Unlike SVM, KNN, and decision tree approaches, RFC can accept missing values. The lengthiest training duration and more complexity are random forest's drawbacks. Boosted trees, which use clone techniques like decision trees, random forests, and bagging, have an effective prediction capability and can defeat this strategy. One reliable method of lowering over-fitting is to boost. The approach depends unduly on outliers. The procedure is almost impossible to scale up, which is another drawback. To overcome the drawbacks of boosting, we suggest an alternative classifier known as an AI Neural Network, which has the advantages of a decentralized memory, the capacity to function with little prior knowledge, and the drawback of being challenging to illustrate. The hybridization of the classifiers is an additional method of illness diagnosis.

- **Benefits of ML**
  - Easily recognizes patterns and trends: Large data sets can be sorted through by machine learning to find patterns and trends that people might miss.
  - Automation: Requires no human intervention: One highly useful feature of machine learning is its capacity to automate various decision-making processes.
  - Continuous Improvement: As machine learning techniques acquire more expertise, their efficacy and precision rise. Computers get more adept at making predictions faster and with more accuracy.
  - Managing data that is multidimensional and multivariate: A multitude of factors influence the dependability of machine learning. Among them is data management. Machine learning is currently the most significant factor in data. Any type of data can be handled by it.

- Wide Applications: Applications for machine learning are numerous. As a result, ML can be used in any of the core fields. Among other industries, machine learning finds application in the medical field.

- **Deep Learning**

Robots can learn to understand by imitating human behaviour through a technique called deep learning in machine learning. Through deep learning, a computer paradigm gains the ability to perform grouping tasks directly from text, audio, or images.

Types of deep learning:

- Radial basis function neural networks
- Feed forward neural network
- Convolution neural network (CNN)
- Multi-layer perceptron
- Modular neural network
- Recurrent neural network

2.1.2. Cervical Cancer Statistical Metrics Worldwide

Significant variations exist in the frequency and death rates of cervical cancer across distinctive countries, according to the World Health Organization (WHO), which provides information on the disease's incidence rates in 2020. Occurs globally in around 604,121 cases, with a death rate of 341,831 compared to other cancer types. Many women lost their lives to cervical cancer; 9 out of 10 deaths occur in low-income countries, while one out of ten occurs in high-income countries.

275,000 women globally lost their lives to cervical cancer in 2008. The third greatest cause of mortality for women worldwide. Of these deaths, 165,810 occurred in Asian countries and 88% occurred in developing nations. It's common to hear people refer to cervical cancer as a unique sickness.

The research indicates that Africa has a high fatality rate. With the successful use of a full suite of HPV antibodies, treatment, and expectation, Australia is expected to have the lowest death rate from cervical cancer. Globally, In 2012, there were about 500,000 instances of cervical cancer reported. In half of these cases, someone died. Approximately 700 people worldwide lose their lives to cervical cancer every day.

These numbers seem to be rising; by 2030, it is predicted that there will be 400,000 deaths annually. Age-adjusted incidence rates (AAIRs) per 110,030 individuals are computed for cancer incidence based on the world population standard.

The following 2018 predictions can be used to gauge the WHO Global Initiative's lofty goal of eliminating cervical cancer as a nation health issue in every nation on the earth. According to estimates from the National Cancer Institute, more than 12,100 women had a cervical cancer diagnosis in 2015. It's possible that 4,000 of them died because of ignorance and disdain for regular checkups and screening procedures.

Cervical Cancer in India

Asia has the greatest fatality rate from cervical cancer, with numerous instances reported there. Cervical cancer affects one in every fifty women worldwide, with India having the greatest incidence of the disease. The world's second-largest population is found in India. More Indian women are researching cervical cancer than any other cancer. However, the incidence rate has risen from 8.8 to this current level. To 11.1 of the group's 200,000 women today.

Cervical cancer is a potential threat to 446.86 million women worldwide who are fifteen years of age or older. Every year, 1,24,844 women are affected by cervical cancer, and 67477 of them pass away from the illness. Ages 15 to 44 are the most common for women to develop cervical cancer. In India, 72,825 of the 26.7% of women who receive a cervical cancer diagnosis each year also pass away from the illness.

A major cause of countless deaths and destruction, Naïven India, 200 women lose their lives to cervical cancer each year, despite 32,000 people receiving a diagnosis. In Uttar Pradesh, 18,682 cases were reported in 2012 compared to 17,368 cases in 2009. After Uttar Pradesh, cervical cancer in 2012 were West Bengal (8396), Andhra Pradesh (7907), Maharashtra (9892), Tamil Nadu (7077), Bihar (9824), and others. By immunizing all young girls against HPVs and keeping an eye out for and treating female illnesses, cervical cancer can be averted. In addition, when detected and treated early, cervical cancer is manageable and may even be cured.

Although the HPV vaccination has a 95% effectiveness rate in reducing the illness, we are unsure of how to assist those who have already had the shot. Doctors advise that even individuals who have received the HPV vaccination should have regular monitoring because there is no guarantee that the recipient will be protected for an extended period of time. Reports state that thirty present of vaccinated people may become unwell again, requiring regular monitoring and biopsies.

2.2. RELATED WORKS

Gathering basic information about current research subjects and methodology is the main objective of conducting a literature review. The research for this thesis describes to diagnose the illness, the study used a variety of deep learning and machine learning methods. Books, journals, and internet resources were among the easily accessible sources used to complete the literature study.

Siegel et al. (2022) Proposed, the Incidence data (up to 2018) were gathered from Over the previous ten years, the proportion of prostate cancer cases detected at an advanced stage increased from 3.9% to 8.2%. However, the incidence of advanced lung cancer cases has sharply decreased, despite a 4.5% annual increase in rates for localized-stage lung cancer. Three-year relative survival rates improved from 21% to 31% because of the increase in the number of localized-stage diagnoses, which rose from 17% in 2004 to 28% in 2018.

The patterns of mortality follow the trends in incidence; lung cancer shows faster reductions, breast cancer progresses more slowly, and prostate cancer stabilizes. As a result of modifications to medical procedures pertaining to screening and treatment, progress has resumed in the case of lung cancer, but it has stagnated in the case of breast and prostate cancers. More funding for early detection and treatment as well as improved targeted cancer control strategies may contribute to a further decline in cancer mortality.

Adweb et al. (2021) Proposed, the goal of identifying cervical cancer using colposcopy pictures. The ReLU activation function network, on the other hand, produced lesser accuracy than Leaky-ReLU and PreLU activation functions were used by the networks. Furthermore, poor generalization results from the ReLU-ResNet architecture's inability to extract the pertinent and intricate properties that differentiate the two cervical classes. As a result, three residual networks were created that had the same design but distinct activation functions. A dataset of colposcopy cervical images was used to train and evaluate the models, and the results (Leaky-RELU and PRELU). Based on experimental results, all built networks were able to identify cervical cancer with high accuracy. The reason behind their enhanced performance is primarily their capacity to tackle the issue of the "dying ReLU" that is linked to the conventional ReLU activation function. Both activation functions demonstrated comparable accuracy, obtaining 90.2% and 100%, respectively.

Yu et al. (2021) Proposed the second model improved upon the first (CNN + SPP). The inception module took the role of the CNN layers in the third model (CNN + Inception). The SPP Layer and inception module were integrated with the original CNN structure in the fourth model, which was named CNN + Inception + SPP. This method worked well for both the Papanicolaou smear test and the ThinPrep cytology tests (TCT). The same testing data and assessment metrics were used to compare and assess the four models' results. According to test findings, the fourth model outperformed the others, with an AUC of 0.997.

Bhavani & Govardhan (2021) proposed, In order to predict cervical cancer from a variety of risk factors, they used SMOTE and Random Forest with RFE and Random Forest with Random Forest for feature extraction. They were able to predict cervical cancer with higher accuracy than the previous method using a stacked ensemble strategy that uses heterogeneous base learners and a meta learner. The experiment's shortcoming is that only one target variable, Biopsy, was taken into consideration. In the future, improved strategies for imputation of missing information should be employed instead of the simplistic imputation methodology we used in this study. In order to prevent type II mistakes, several data balancing techniques were also used, bearing in mind that these algorithms are simpler and take less time to compute than alternative approaches.

According to **Lavanya Devi et al. (2021)**, a novel automated cervical cancer diagnosis technique was created by merging PCA with fuzzy C-means tailored for the disease. Pap smear images are classified into clear KNN classification and k fold cross validation. The outcomes of the suggested approach are contrasted with those of Ensemble Bagged Trees, Linear Discriminant Analysis, and Fine Gaussian SVM. The effectiveness is evaluated using metrics such as the F1 - score, precision, sensitivity, average accuracy, specificity, minimum accuracy, and maximum accuracy. With an accuracy of 94.86%, a greatest accuracy 96.28%, and a minimum accuracy 94.15%, three-fold cross-validation demonstrates the excellent performance of the proposed method. Additionally, the results display an accuracy 96.31%, sensitivity 97.96%, specificity 83.65%, and F1-score 96.87%.

A novel approach to integrating CRF and CNN into a fully trainable architecture was put out by **Soni & Soni (2021)**. The fundamental concept is to copy the regularisation characteristics of an actual CRF optimizer using a custom module. This module is trained using samples produced by a CRF optimizer and employs a conventional CNN architecture. If a good CRF optimizer is utilized, the ground truth can be recovered indefinitely without the user's involvement. Our approach has an advantage over earlier research in that it eliminates the need to incorporate the challenging physics of optimizing CRF into CNN. CNN – CRF provides a variety of applications for evaluating and capturing images of the internal anatomy of the human body. Neural networks and CT scans are two examples of the numerous types of medical pictures that may be analyzed with the help of machine learning algorithms. Medical image analysis has benefited greatly from machine learning. An experiment shows that the CNN-CRF strategy beats the CNN method.

Tripathi et al, (2021) proposed, deep learning techniques for classification were used to the SIPAKMED papsmear picture dataset as a baseline for evaluating future classification strategies. The given source provided the publicly available dataset, which was then separated into training and testing subsets. By training the model on the target dataset, the pre-trained model parameters were fine-tuned. This dataset is more relevant than many other datasets used in previously published research because it takes into account all of the genetic and environmental changes that have happened over the last decade. Parabasal, Koilocytotic, Dyskeratotic, Superficial-intermediate, and Metaplastic were the five categorization categories. ResNet-152 was found to have the best performance among the classifiers. The classifications still have a lot of room for improvement. All of these discoveries are limited to a specific dataset's visual features. The ResNet-152 architecture achieved the highest accuracy of 94.89%.

In order to classify and forecast cervical cancer, **Khamparia et al. (2021)** suggested a computer vision system that uses a hybrid convolutional and variational encoder deep learning methodology. Deep convolutional networks, which have been further optimized for accuracy, are used to extract the features. Of the 917 pap smear cells of the malignant image type, 90% (642) were used for training, while the remaining 30% were used for testing. The variational auto encoder is trained using the softmax layer, which minimizes the results. Using different epochs, the suggested design obtained variational accuracy of 99.2 percent with a 2*2 filter size and 99.4 percent with a 3*3 filter size. In the initial diagnosis of cervical cancer, the suggested hybrid variational convolutional auto encoder method outperformed popular machine learning techniques.

Ali et al. (2021) proposed, a useful ML based classification algorithm that uses clinical datasets to diagnose cervical cancer in its early stages. Four main categories of attributes were present in the Kaggle data repository CC dataset that we used: Hinselmann, Schiller, biopsy and cytology. Following data extraction from public repositories, the dataset was pre-processed and transformed using multiple FT approaches to reform the dataset after it was divided into classes. The dataset was then run through five various kinds of classifiers (RF, Kstar, RT SPAARC, and Ibk) to determine their performance characteristics. Three feature transformation techniques were applied to these datasets: Z-score normalization, sine function, and log transformation. It was evaluated how well different supervised machine learning techniques performed in terms of classification. For both the biopsy and cytology data, the Random Forest (RF) model achieved an accuracy of 98.33% and 98.65%, respectively. The Tree (RT) method was the most effective strategy; RF and IBK were the best approaches for Schiller (98.58 percent) and Hinselmann (99.16 percent), respectively. The logarithmic feature transformation approach performed best for biopsy datasets. The findings of this research show that proper categorization may effectively and efficiently diagnose CC in its early stages.

A cervical cancer detection approach based on the random forest regression method was proposed by **Gupta & Hasija (2021)**. Unlike other studies that concentrate on accuracy and precision, this work looks at the recall-based technique and its benefits over earlier methods. Himmelmann's test, cytology, biopsy, and Schiller's test are the four diagnostic procedures used to identify cervical cancer early. Each test is analyzed independently, and the confusion matrix curve (ROC), receiver operator, and recall score are used to analyze the results. The fast increase in new instances strains an already overburdened medical and clinical diagnosis system, and chronic diseases like cervical cancer have significant repercussions for patients as well as society.

Xia et al. (2020) developed a Series parallel fusion network as a novel network topology for detecting cervical cancer cells (SPFNet). The researchers developed an SPFNet by enhancing a conventional deep learning classification network, making it more suitable for object identification tasks. Unlike traditional frameworks that rely on classification networks as their strength, our series module features five distinct head components designed to optimize the network topology for specific detection tasks. The experimental findings reveal that our detection framework outperforms all others in terms of generating optimal outcomes.

Huang et al. (2020) Proposed, for classifying cervical biopsy tissue images. While retaining classification accuracy, Feature selection and serial fusion utilizing the LASSO technique resulted in a 35.87 second reduction in the average optimization time. A total of 468 images of tumor tissue were identified and categorized using the EL-SVM classifier. A curve was used to assess the classifier's capacity for generalization. A study of experimental results indicates that 99.64 percent of cervical cancer cases and 99.64 precent of low-grade squamous intraepithelial cancer cases could be classified as normal. A classification accuracy of 84.25 precent was achieved for normal-high-grade squamous intraepithelial lesions (LSIL). Based on the results of (HSIL) categorization, 87.34% was efficient, 76.34 precent was efficient, 91.88 precent was accurate, and 81.54 percent accuracy was achieved by HSIL- cervical cancer classification.

Li et al. (2020) proposed, a deep learning (DL) method for accurately identifying LSIL+ using time-lapsed colposcopic pictures of cervical cancer. DL nets are used by the software to extract features from each of a patient's colposcopic pictures individually. Feature Fusion Nets and Key-frame feature encoding networks are the two fundamental components of the suggested scheme. The characteristics of the colposcopic images and original picture are acquired at during the acetic acid test, the 60s, 90s, 120s, and 150s were encoded using feature encoding networks. The suggested architecture is tested using large scale cervical dataset that includes pictures from 7,668 patients. Colposcopists can also compete utilising our computer-assisted diagnostic approach. As a result of the trial, with a classification accuracy of 78.33%, the deep learning system matches the performance of expert colposcopists.

Jia et al. (2020) proposed a CNN in conjunction with robust features obtained using Gabor and Gray-Level Co-occurrence Matrix (GLCM) as a novel framework for constructing the basis of powerful features that efficiently categorize cervical cells. These combined features were then used to classify data using a SVM. To increase the model's durability, an effective technique for data augmentation was developed. On two different datasets, the metrics of specificity, sensitivity, and accuracy were used to test the proposed approach. Our suggested approach beat baselines and state-of-the-art models for 2-class identification in the mass, with Sn, Sp, and Acc of 98.9, 99.4, and 99.3 respectively. The outcomes showed how useful the CNN-SVM model with its deep features may be for classifying cells in the early detection of cervical cancer. Additionally, the approach outlined in this study demonstrated the efficacy of our method in identifying malignant cells by performing well in the classification of positive cells.

Ghoneim et al. (2020) suggested a convolutional neural network (CNN) for system categorization and cervical cancer cell identification. Either an AE-based classifier or an ELM-based classifier was used once the CNN model was included into the system. To recover deeply learnt attributes, cell pictures were fed into the CNN model. Both fine-tuning and transfer learning were used in the CNN model's implementation. As an alternative to the ELM, classifiers based on auto encoders and multi-layer perceptrons (MLP) were investigated. Using the Herlev database, the study looked at both deep and shallow CNN models. 99.7% accuracy in the two-class challenge and 97.2% accuracy in the seven - class problem was attained by the ELM-based classifier.

Luo et al. (2020) Suggested the method divides the training data into predefined classes using the k-means algorithm during data pre-processing. These classes are then combined for testing to improve the model's generalization capacity. The vital idea behind the method is to combine features from different network architectures and optimize the small dataset in order to achieve integration on both the data and structural levels. When compared to senior physicians utilizing a sample of 100 tests, it revealed considerable gains in diagnostic performance and efficiency. Then, based on the transfer learning, two types of CNN are finetuned independently, and the XGBoost technique is utilised to merge the diverse CNN decision outcomes for maximising the final prediction. Simultaneously, depending on the integration of the 2 approaches, two integration techniques (inner-to-outer and outer-to-inner) are devised for the result. Neural network training can be improved by combining the K-means data preparation method with the suggested multi-decision feature fusion strategy. Furthermore, in order to meet clinical diagnostic needs, the proposed K-means data pre-processing technique can enhance computer-aided diagnosis findings.

Wang et al. (2020) proposed, an adaptive pruning deep transfer learning-based automated CAD cervical smear image categorization system. Use of the PsiNet-TAP system is recommended. The result is a more broadly applicable pre-trained model compared to a scratch-built model. We investigate the effects of hierarchy, filters, and feature maps using the pruning criterion and loss function, doing adaptive pruning to produce a more effective model. To create the pre-trained model, we used transfer learning since the number of photographs was limited. In addition, the convolution layer was adjusted, and various kernels that interfered with classification were removed. We can improve cervical cancer detection, notably by distinguishing aberrant from cyto-pathologically normal-appearing cell images. PsiNet-TAP, the suggested method, was assessed using 389 pictures from cervical Pap smears. The strategy has shown incredible accuracy (more than 98 percent), indicating the potential of the recommended.

Asyhar et al. (2020) proposed, using colposcopy data and the LSTM algorithm, cervical cancer can be detected. After pre-processing, which involved normalizing pixel intensity, eliminating noise, and altering the colposcopy image data based on grey levels, the LSTM algorithm was used to detect cervical cancer. The information will be turned into spatial information with pre-processing, which is known as the reshaping process. The LSTM algorithm will be used to classify the vector data created by the reshaping process. Using computational LSTM computations, the accuracy of colposcopy test findings can be enhanced. Computational calculations, in addition to improving efficiency, make it much easier for humans to diagnose cervical cancer. The amount of hidden layers in the classifier employing 150 hidden layers is the ideal amount for classifying colposcopy data using the LSTM algorithm with a 66 present accuracy.

Saini et al. (2020) proposed a deep-learning-based system based on colposcopy pictures has been presented, which can aid doctors in medication planning and follow-up therapy. The DenseNet model was used to inspire the architecture of the suggested technique, ColpoNet, Compared to previous models, this method is computationally more efficient. Additionally, it has been assessed and verified against a number of alternative techniques using a dataset that was made available by the National Cancer Institute. VGG16, LeNet, ResNet50, GoogleNet, and AlexNet are examples of deep-learning models that may be used to test the breadth of their application. ColpoNet had the greatest performance rate, with an accuracy of 81.353 precent, according to the experimental research. In comparison to other cutting-edge deep methods A categorization system like this might be used in clinics to improve patient care. Furthermore, the suggested technique has certain limitations in terms of picture segmentation and pre-processing processes for identifying ROI, thus accuracy may be improved by focusing solely on relevant data.

Kudva et al. (2020) proposed the starting strengths of the filters were derived from pre trained VGG-16 and AlexNet nets that emphasise the acetowhite characteristics in two shallow layer CNNs. These nets were used to categorise photos of the cervix. It has a 91.46 present classification overall accuracy. The most filters in the convolution layer that emphasise the margin of acetowhite areas and texture inside the acetowhite area may enhance the network's effectiveness. Using AlexNet and the VGG-16, a CNN is built and trained from the ground up, identifying only the filters' beginning values that are relevant. This research included 2198 cervix pictures, 1090 of which were abnormal, and of which were positive. The efficiency of our hybrid domain adaptation experiment was 91.46 precent increased than existing techniques.

Cervical cancer is one of the most common gynecologic malignancies worldwide, according to **Lu & Alrashoud (2020)**. Cervical cancer is a largely preventable disease, and the best method to reduce its worldwide burden is by early screening. Regrettably, little awareness, restricted access to medical facilities, and expensive treatments prohibit needy communities in developing nations from getting regular checkups. The aim of this study is to use a novel ensemble approach to predict the risk of cervical cancer. To address the difficulties encountered in earlier cervical cancer research, this approach makes use of a voting strategy. A data rectification approach is presented to improve prediction performance. Furthermore, as an optional approach, a gene-assistance module is offered to bolster the predictions' resilience. Several analyses of the suggested method are carried out, and the findings show that the voting procedure can be used to precisely estimate the risk of acquiring cervical cancer. The suggested solution is more workable and scalable than alternative approaches.

Singh & Goyal (2020) proposed, online and offline machine learning methods such as, Gaussian Nave Bayes, Gradient Boosting, K-Nearest Neighbor, Decision Tree and Logistic Regression for two-class problem for identification of cervical cancer. This paper also uses hybrid strategies to solve the difficult of segmentation and optimises the number of features by employing additional tree classifiers. The use of hybrid segmentation algorithms for segmenting Pap smear pictures in cytoplasm, background, and nucleus, as well as the selection of most significant characteristics using an extra tree classifier, has established a lot of attention. On the basis of performance indicators and CPU time, many machine learning methods have been reviewed. The highest level of accuracy reached was 100 percent, demonstrating the importance of ML algorithms in the detection of cervical cancer. Furthermore, numerous algorithms have precision, recall, and F1 scores of 100 percent or above, indicating that this work is reliable.

Win et al. (2020) proposed, a Pap smear pictures, Image capture, classification, feature selection, feature extraction, cell segmentation, and image enhancement were the six processes in our suggested system. Our suggested approach first segmented each individual cell component, such as the cytoplasm and nucleus, and then used a machine learning based technique to determine if the cells were malignant or not. In the past, a number of strategies in this direction have been offered. However, the precision has not been discovered to be easily accessible. As a feature selection method, the RF (random forest) algorithm was applied. Five classifiers were used in the classification step: SVM, boosted trees, bagged trees, LD, and KNN. The seven-class and five-class multi-class problems had respective percentages of 90.84% and 94.09%., while for the two-class problem it was 98.47% and 98.27%. The key benefit of our suggested strategy is that it improves the predictive performance in distinguishing aberrant from normal cells.

Using pap smear image analysis, **Hussain et al. (2020)** suggested a DL method to assist a pathologist in automated and quick diagnostic prediction. This study examines six deep convolutional neural network architectures for the multi-class detection of cervical precancerous and malignant lesions: GoogleNet, ResNet (ResNet-50 and ResNet-101), VGGNet (VGG-16 and VGG-19), and AlexNet. This article demonstrates how pathologists can use deep learning to enable automatic and quick diagnosis predictions using Pap smear picture analysis. This technique, in contrast to conventional ones, corrects errors and does away with the requirement for segmentation or human feature extraction. The best results (0.989 accuracy, 0.979 specificity, and 0.978 sensitivity).

Susan & Subashini (2019) proposed, a web portal for rural women in taking up the screening examine for cervical cancer. The patient and doctors will have access to a web portal through which they will be authenticated. It comprises a patient's clinical narrative and a doctor's assessment, as well as the actual MobileODT cervix screening image and the data obtained and reviewed. Filters such as the median filter and average filter are used in the suggested image analysis model's denonising procedure. This enables clinicians to efficiently analyse the screened image in the final analysis. The experiment is carried out with a real time cervix image, and the results show that it is effective.

Karim and Neehal (2019) suggested using SVM as the base classifier in ensemble approaches to improve illness detection accuracy. Ensemble approaches were applied to the algorithm that performed the best in order to increase overall accuracy. It will remain an option since nature-inspired optimization algorithms can be used to further improve its precision. With a 98.12% accuracy rate, the ensemble technique with Bagging methodology achieved extraordinarily high precision, recall, and f-measure values.

According to **Ojha et al. (2019)**, a questionnaire that asks about a person's sexual activity can be used to identify HPV infection, which is the leading cause of cervical cancer, by using a number of machine learning methodologies. It also seeks to identify the stage of cervical intra – epithelial neoplasia in order to facilitate early diagnosis and therapy and stop the development of cervical cancer. In the second stage of image analysis, eliminate the three essential features for detection and evaluate their precision by classifying the data using eight machine learning techniques. The classifiers that achieve the highest accuracy with the given dataset are Decision Tree, Gaussian Naive

Bayes, Support Vector Classifier, and Quadratic Discriminant Analysis. Among the best are classifiers with 100% sensitivity.

Liu et al. (2019) proposed, a new fuzzy reasoning model for CIN categorization that uses both grayscale and textural aspects of the aceto white area during an acetic-acid test. Here 505 patients had their photos examined before and after the acetic acid test. To extract the acetowhite zone, an artificial picture segmentation method was used. The CIN index was created using fuzzy reasoning that took into account expert knowledge. For three individual traits, the averaged sensitivity was 80.8 percent, 80.9 percent, and 82.8 percent, while the mean specificity was 82.0 percent, 87.4 percent, and 86.2 percent, respectively. In terms of precision, image texture attributes exceeded temporal grayscale change. Combining texture-based and grayscale characteristics might result in a synergistic effect that improves overall classification performance. The suggested fuzzy reasoning approach might improve sensitivity much further without adding any new features. In the future, the automatic CIN categorization method put forth here may prove to be a useful screening aid. Cervical cancer prevention has received a lot of consideration recently.

Johnes Obungoloch et al. (2019) proposed, Based on Pap smear pictures, this study proposes an automated system for the diagnosis and classification of cervical cancer. Fuzzy C-means was used for classification, and a Simulink model with a wrapper filter was used for feature selection. The study concludes with conclusions and assessments of the findings. Three distinct techniques were used to assess the classifier, and the results showed accuracies of 98.88%, 99.28%, and 97.47% for each dataset, respectively. By carefully selecting cell features that boosted segmentation outcomes and the amount of groups employed, a comprehensive feature extraction strategy increased defuzzification and classification performance. Applying the approach to the Herlev benchmark Pap smear dataset produced specificity of 97.47%, accuracy of 98.88%, and sensitivity of 99.28%, outperforming numerous other systems. Clinical laboratory Pap smear slides were used to get these results.

William et al. (2019) proposed, a computer assisted diagnosis tool to improve the reliability and accuracy of the PAP test. The invention of a technique for automatic classification and diagnosis of cervical cancer using pap-smear images is described in this work. A Weka Segmentation classifier was utilised to segment the scene, and a sequential reduction technique was used for material rejection. By removing instances that are obviously benign, this technology's main benefit in a cervical cancer screening workflow is its capacity to shorten the time cytotechnicians spend screening a large number of Pap smears. The suggested method may assess a complete Pap smear slide in approximately three minutes, compared to the five to ten minutes that manual examination usually takes per slide. This method beats a number of current algorithms by obtaining specificity of 97.47%, accuracy of 98.88%, and sensitivity of 99.28%. When applied to pap-smear slides from a pathological lab classification error, false negative rate and the false positive rate were 5.00 percent, 10.10 percent and, 0.01 percent respectively.

Kanitkar et al. (2019) suggested, a method for detecting cervical anomalies using Machine Learning (ML) instead of imaging data are presented. The new population data machine learning model may be the answer to low-cost cervical screening in rural regions, depending on the outputs of the machine learning technique, allowing patients to undergo more expensive screening tests such as Pap smear and biopsy. As can be seen from the findings, ANN outperforms all of the other algorithms. Furthermore, the findings show that factors such as menstrual history, menopause and education level status have a substantial impact on predicting cervical abnormalities in patients.

Alam and associates (2019) Decision tree algorithms and other data mining approaches are used in the suggested predictive analysis. A 10 fold cross validation process was used to validate the results, and the improved decision tree performed the best. Using the Hinslemann screening method, the boosted decision tree achieved an excellent prediction score of 0.978 on the AUROC curve, outperforming earlier classifiers. Utilizing the growing amount of patient data on the disease and the rapidly evolving analytical technologies, we aim to identify the best effective screening approach for patients with cervical cancer in order to enhance patient treatment.

A low-cost visual screening method was intended by **Gerbino et al. (2019)** to identify cervical cancer in its early stages. Our goal is to provide an inexpensive visual screening technique for the early diagnosis of cervical cancer. By creating a minimally invasive, affordable system that would enable women in certain circumstances to be checked for the disease, this technique aims to increase the identification of cervical cancer. Because it prevents oxygen diffusion and supports anaerobic culture while allowing for easy observation and manipulation by the client, this form was chosen as the best option for the device. Women in limited situations rarely have access to pap smears, which help in early detection in developed countries.

Lidiya Thampi & Varghese Paul (2018) Proposed the analyses and summarizes numerous methodologies used in evaluating digital cervical pictures and underlines the accompanying issues. In both males and females, the most common viral infection caused by unprotected sexual contact is the human papillomavirus (HPV), which is widely distributed. Nearly 25% of all female cancers are cervical cancers, making it one of the most dangerous health problems for women in impoverished nations like India. In contemporary healthcare, a number of sophisticated methods and instruments have been developed for the early detection of cervical cancer. Notably, the incidence rate of cervical cancer has dropped dramatically by roughly 50% to 66% since the advent of the Papanicolaou smear, the Pap test is another name for it. However, problems like uneven staining, cell overlap, and poor image quality make cervical cell nuclei difficult to segment.

Zheng Hu & Ding Ma (2018) proposed, Cervical cancer is the 3rd most frequent cancer in women globally, and our understanding of its prevention and treatment is constantly changing. Cervical cancer is largely caused by the HPV, yet it's vital to remember that HPV infection does not cause the disease directly. The majority of HPV infections are temporary, and the host's immune system can eradicate them on their own, so HPV-related cancer is a comparatively uncommon consequence. In actuality, cervical cancer frequently takes decades to manifest after a persistent HPV infection. We examine the main drivers of HPV persistence and cervical carcinogenesis in this review, along with new ideas and innovations in cancer treatment. Above all, we address how these developments may open the door to clinical precision medicine, which will provide patients with early diagnosis, prevention, and treatment plans.

Karthiga Jaya & Senthil Kumar (2018) proposed, Cervical cancer is identified and classified using an ANFIS (Adaptive Network-based Fuzzy Inference System) classifier in this method. The picture 30arlier30v, edge detection, classification, and segmentation phases make up the suggested system. Fast Fourier Transforms are used to register images (FFTs). Grey Level and Trinary Features, along with the Grey Level Co-occurrence Matrix (GLCM), are extracted after the cervical image has been validated. The ANFIS classifier is then used to train and classify these recovered features. The categorized cervical image is subjected to transformation techniques in order to detect and segment cancer. Research has indicated that the suggested methodology surpasses current approaches concerning precision,31arlier31veness, and discrimination.

Arya et al. (2018) proposed, a simple cytology test used to identify cancer early is called a Pap smear. To acquire optimal findings from the Pap smear, the expertise of qualified pathologists is necessary. However, pathologists are not as readily available in India as they should be, especially in rural regions. Several texture-based features are presented in this paper to extract meaningful and instructive aspects from single-cell images. To help identify the outlines of the nucleus and cytoplasm, textural features are extracted using first-order histogram, LBP, GLCM, Laws, and DWT. Based on the trained characteristics, single-cell pictures are classified as either normal or malignant using ANN and SVM. Both single features and feature combinations are treated with these techniques. The combined feature set yields the best outcomes. The generated MNITJ dataset, which consists of 330 single cervical cell pictures, and the publically accessible Herlev benchmark dataset are used to assess the system. According to experimental data, the suggested texture-based features perform much better in terms of accuracy in cervical cancer detection than conventional shape-based features.

Deng et al. (2018) developed three different techniques of ML are utilised to classify the UCI cervical cancer dataset. The dataset consists of four target variables (Hinselmann, Schiller, Biopsy, & Cytology) and 32 risk factors. In order to address the imbalance in the dataset before to classification, the Borderline-SMOTE method was utilized. Upon analyzing the outcomes of classifications based on many criteria, it was discovered that Random Forest and XGBoost outperform SVM in the diagnosis of benign and malignant tumors. Both approaches exhibit superior accuracy along with great sensitivity and specificity. Furthermore, we discovered five major risk variables: age, number of sensual partners, usage of hormonal contraception, number of pregnancies and age at first sexual contact. These factors have a considerable impact on the diagnosis of cervical cancer.

Yamuna Devi et al. (2018) suggested, an ideal classification strategy for cancer detection is offered by this method. First, noise reduction is applied to the image in order to remove any unnecessary noise. The boundaries of the image are then defined via image refinement. To separate the image into discrete regions, two segmentation techniques are applied: threshold segmentation and watershed segmentation. This pixel grouping technique works especially well since the threshold value acts as the primary selection criterion, converting grayscale images to binary representation. To separate the tumor components from the image, watershed segmentation is applied, and the resulting segments are then thresholded. The multiclass categorization stage of the suggested technique then makes use of these properties. A multiclass support vector machine (SVM) is used to diagnose tumors; estimations indicate that 80–90% of malignancies may be correctly categorized using this classifier. While recognizing tumorous regions in medical imaging is a difficult process, the suggested approach successfully locates the affected areas.

The Random Forest (RF) classification approach and the synthetic minority oversampling strategy were proposed by **Abdoh et al. (2018).** SMOTE is utilized to solve this issue because of the imbalance in the data set that was used. The data set includes four target variables (Hinselmann, Schiller, Cytology, and Biopsy) and 32 risk factors. According to our research, employing SMOTE enhances overall classification performance whereas utilizing a typical classification strategy decreases it. According to our results, the SMOTE-RF model performs better in terms of accuracy, specificity, and PPA than the SVM classification method. We found that RFE and PCA may be utilized to properly diagnose patients with cervical cancer after comparing the results of our studies. The SMOTE-RF, which possessed every characteristic of every cervical cancer test, outperformed them, nonetheless.

A deep learning-based approach to cervical cancer screening was proposed by **Taha et al. (2017)**. Instead of building and training a convolutional neural network (CNN) from scratch, use a Support Vector Machine (SVM) classifier. Using this new approach, we applied a standard SVM classifier after first extracting features using the pre-trained AlexNet architecture. It is possible to optimize the system without spending any money on resources or computing. According to our experimental findings, the suggested methodology for single cell pap smears based on the Herlev public database performs better than the state-of-the-art techniques currently in use.

Sun et al. (2017) proposed, a random forest (RF) classifier with ReliefF feature selection, a system for cervical tumour is given. Twenty features were retrieved using pre-processing, segmentation, and feature extraction. Using ReliefF, 20 characteristics were sorted according to weight during the feature selection step. The RF approach was employed as a classifier in the classification phase, and various dimensions of features were used to train the classifier. The Herlev data set, obtained at Herlev University Hospital, was utilised to test the efficacy of the suggested technique, with Pap smear pictures classified into two categories: normal and abnormal. After a 10-fold cross validation, the experimental findings revealed that the top 13 features based on the RF classifier provided the greatest classification performance, outperforming C4.5, Logistic Regression, and Naive Bayes. The AUC value was 0.9804, and the accuracy was 94.44 percent. The findings also supported the use of cytoplasmic characteristics in categorization.

Wu et al. (2017) proposed two sophisticated Support Vector Machine (SVM) techniques are proposed for the diagnosis of cervical cancer samples: The improvement of malignant cancer sample detection is the goal of these techniques. When compared to the normal SVM, SVM-PCA and SVM-RFE may both achieve comparable performance with fewer features. SVM-PCA and SVM-RFE, in particular, have the capacity to decrease feature counts from 30 to 8 in order to complete the classification. Cervical cancer data can be derived from cytology, biopsy, Schiller, and Hinselmann. The three SVM-based techniques have successfully identified and categorised all four targets. Following that, we do a comparison between these three approaches and compare our risk factor ranking result to the ground reality. The problem can be efficiently solved using SVM-PCA and SVM RFE. With the same amount of features as SVM-RFE, SVM-PCA has a greater capacity.

Unlersen et al. (2017) proposed, a machine learning techniques for detecting the possibility of cervical cancer by using different techniques like k-Nearest Neighbor, BayesNet and Multilayer Perceptron. Patients were categorised in this research depending on their replies to a questionnaire and see who has a higher risk of cervical cancer. While one key goal in cancer possibility estimate is to maximise the number of accurately categorised instances, another significant goal is to minimise the number of false positive instances. The dataset contains 858 entries with 33 characteristics and a biopsy result for each. There are 55 patients diagnosed with cervical cancer, compared to 803 healthy people. The dataset was split into two groups at random: test and train. The train dataset contains 565 objects, or 66% of the whole dataset. The rest of the data has been labelled as a test dataset. The test dataset has 292 records. As a result, the rates of falsely classified instances are 1.37 percent, 1.71 percent, and 2.05 percent, respectively. Because the amount of properly categorized occurrences for Bayes Net and k-NN methods is so close, false negative outcomes become more important when deciding on the optimal method. According to the authors, the optimum solution for this problem is the k-NN method with 86 neighbours.

Hasan et al. (2017) proposed, a cervical screening intervention programme aimed at encouraging women of all ages to engage in the screening. None has focused on the tailored intervention for cervical cancer screening. This programme could assist women in recognising the risk of cervical cancer. This project is an effort to promote a cervical cancer knowledge reservoir that will assist women in building behaviour, ideas, and ethics that will lead to a successful cervical cancer screening lifestyle. The strategy could benefit the health-care system by lowering cervical cancer death rates and costs. According to preliminary findings, around 96 percent of those who participated in the intervention programme went on to get screened, indicating that a proper intrinsically driven cervical cancer programme is needed.

Vidya et al. (2016) proposed using strong Data Mining methods to identify whether a cervix is normal or malignant in 2016. In the medical field, data mining is crucial for forecasting. This methodology is used to predict if a cervix is benign or malignant using the algorithm, and RFT in conjunction with K-means learning were all used in the study. The accuracy of the CART output was found to be 83.87%. Using MATLAB coding, the Random Forest Tree was used to improve prediction accuracy, and it was able to achieve a prediction accuracy of 93.54%. Furthermore, the RFT-K-means learning strategy achieved a high accuracy of 96.77% since the K-means method works well for processing huge datasets.

Sukumar & Gnanamurthy (2016) proposed, a technique for computer-assisted automated identification and diagnosis of cervical cancer utilising Pap smear images is suggested. The suggested approach is utilised to assess and measure the morphology of cervical cells. Pre-processing, feature extraction, nucleus area segmentation, and classification are all included in the suggested methodology. The nucleus cell region is divided using morphological techniques. Early cervical cancer intervention is made possible by scheduling the patient for a biopsy and subsequent surgical therapy upon the detection of abnormal cells. Cervical dysplastic cell segmentation using the proposed technique shows 98.74% accuracy, 99.65% specificity, and 92.68% sensitivity.

Meng Zhao et al. (2016) proposed Our solution drastically reduces computing complexity by dividing the image into blocks of a given size, as opposed to segmenting individual cells as is the case with existing methods. Whether or not problematic cells are present in a frame, statistical variables like texture and color can be used to identify significant differences between frames when studied using predictive analytics. These attributes as inputs. 1,100 quasi blocks, of which 110 are suspicious, the model is trained using them. The collected findings indicate that our technique has a reliability of roughly 98.98%. Notably, the accuracy is an astounding 99.33%, and the sensitivity, which is crucial in cancer screening, is 95.0%. Our computational analysis is performed on block images, in contrast to other approaches, which greatly increases processing efficiency by doing away with the requirement for pre-computed analytical tasks. Furthermore, the technique has significant diagnostic value because it naïves based on actual WSCCI data.

Machmud & Wijaya (2016) proposed to determine the probability of Ca - Cervix risk based on behaviour and its determinant, machine learning, Nave Bayes, and Logistic Regression are employed as classifiers. Ca Cervix is a severe public health issue that affects women from the world, but it is luckily avoidable. If discovered early, the primary prevention of Ca Cervix through behaviour prevention since early identification has several benefits, including reduced mortality and increased treatment efficacy. The models in this study are promising based on the experimental results, since they have a classification accuracy of over 90% and an AUC of over 0.95. Because we present both accuracy and AUC, this study is still experimental and subject to further development. As a result, we create a standard for future research comparisons.

Paul et al. (2015) suggested using Pap smear pictures to automatically diagnose cervical cancer. This method uses a bi-group enhancer to separate nuclei pixels from other object pixels after removing impulse noise from Pap smear images using an adaptive median filter. Next, segmentation techniques are used to separate the nucleus areas from the cervical smear images. During the technique's classification phase, the Pap smear cervical cell images were separated into normal and abnormal cells using a minimum distance classifier and a K-nearest neighbor classifier. The minimal distance classifier has a classification accuracy of 92.37 percent in distinguishing between normal and diseased cells. K-nearest neighbour, on the other hand, has a remarkable accuracy of 98.31%. The detecting technique's efficiency is 92.37 percent for minimum distance classifications and 98.31 percent for K-nearest neighbour classifications, respectfully.

Nithin et al. (2015) suggested an automated technique for identifying cervical cancer based on spectrum received from a photonic crystal based biosensor in 2015. A photonic crystal-based electrical and magnetic dielectric constant sensor that is extremely sensitive to changes in the dielectric constant for a set of current concentration levels in a static environment under the impact of electromagnetic radiation ranging from UV to IR. By precisely determining the refractive index of each kind, the sensor can distinguish between cervical malignant tissue and normal tissue. We developed a MATLAB programme that extracts and classifies the features of the sensor's output automatically. The associated sensor data is fed into a machine learning technique called a Naive Bayesian classifier, which uses automatically generated features to distinguish between normal and malignant tissue spectra. A photonic crystal-based biosensor that incorporates sensor data and an automatic classification archive increases cervical cancer diagnosis. As a result, the automated method, which combines both sensors and automatic categorization, can be utilised to identify cervical cancer more effectively and accurately.

Bountris et al. (2015) proposed, a decision support system based on an ensemble of Random Forests (RFs) for the cognitive combining of the findings of conventional and supplementary approaches for Cervical cancer diagnosis, on demand to maximise the advantages of each method and provide more accurate results. The suggested ensemble of Random Forests produced encouraging results proposed that this strategy might increase diagnostic accuracy and help the management of women with aberrant cervical cancer screening data. Furthermore, when compared to other approaches, the suggested architecture has many benefits and appears to be more appropriate for the application, as: a) It enables us to evaluate situations in which examinations are missing, including pap tests, and it may offer precise risk estimations for the development of CIN. The recommended method has good overall accuracy (91.8%), specificity (93.3%), and sensitivity (86.1%) in diagnosing.

Song et al. (2015) proposed, An MSCN-based approach and graph partitioning are described for the segmentation of cervical cytoplasm and nuclei. Deep learning is used to extract scale invariant characteristics and then segment areas centred at each pixel using the MSCN. An automatic graph partitioning approach based on the pretrained feature refines the coarse segmentation. A distinct border, which is then used to create markers to divide touching nuclei. Super-pixel, graph partitioning, and MSCN were found to be extremely successful for cervical cell segmentation in our experiments. The amazing segmentation results show that the suggested technology may be utilised to detect and diagnose cervical cancer automatically. State-of-the-art performance is attained as compared to older algorithms. Furthermore, the suggested technique is a good tool to screen for cervical cancer and offers strong evidence for automated assistance.

Sarwar et al. (2015) proposed the effectiveness of an artificial intelligence-based system for cervical cancer screening using Pap smear image characterisation and categorization. After being stained using the Papanicolaou procedure, a sample of cells is examined under a microscope for any atypical developments that might indicate precancerous or possibly precancerous alterations. If abnormal findings are discovered, they are submitted to more detailed diagnostic subroutines. Cervical abnormalities can be identified by analyzing cell pictures, which enables early intervention and lowers the incidence and death rates of cervical cancer. With its high classification efficiency, the hybrid ensemble approach that has been suggested can help qualified healthcare workers and medical professionals diagnose cervical cancer through Pap smear screening with greater sensitivity and specificity. Outperforming all other algorithms, this hybrid ensemble technique achieved an accuracy of almost 96% for two-class issues and roughly 78% for seven-class problems. Compared to all other solo classifiers, the results for the two-class and seven-class tasks were much better.

Xu et al. (2015) proposed, a cost effective and automated approach that may be used in low-resource areas. Firstly, they propose a much more unique multi-feature description for conveying cervical image data by combining the pyramidal histogram of local binary pattern feature with a current description. Secondly, they use the AdaBoost approach to extract features and develop a binary classifier to distinguish between high-risk and low-risk patient encounters. Our AdaBoost classification may be tweaked to obtain a high level of purity, which is required for clinical usage. Furthermore, the PLBP-PLAB-PHOG multi-feature description is meant to encode colour, edge, shape, and texture information in cervigrams. Our strategy outperforms human judgments on different screening test-based CIN classification and outperforms existing image-based CIN classification algorithms.

Yang & Huang (2014) proposed, a piezoelectric immunosensor for early cervical detection of cancer. The method suggested in this research featured a quick analysing time for detecting p16INK4a, a protein associated to cervical cancer. The p16INK4a antibody was dripped over the centre of the AT-cut crystal, as well as precipitate from several clinical samples. The immunosensor's resonator was shifted when the p16INK4a was absorbed by the antibody, and the resonant frequency was connected to the amount of p16INK4a in the supernatant. This approach has the potential to be a promising assay for detecting the cervical lesions 38arlier. In comparison to other strategies, the one proposed in this study is more objective, speedier, and less reliant on technical knowledge.

Table 2.1 Summary of the papers reviewed

Image acquisition	Pre-processing	Segmentation	Classification
• USE open dataset. • arXiv dataset • ERUDIT • Her lev • MNITJ • PubMed • Datasets from hospitals	• Median filter • Gaussian Filter • Band pass filter	• Adaptive Histogram Equalization • Hough Transformation • Super Pixel Based • Seed Based Region Growing • Markov Random Field • Edge detection	• K-Means • Artificial Neural Networks (ANN) • Support Vector Machines • Fuzzy C-Means • ResNet-152 • Bayesian Networks • K-Nearest Neighbor • Naïve Bayes classifier

Table 2.2 Benefits and Drawbacks of Segmentation Classification Methods

Technique	Advantages	Limitations
1. Segmentation		
Fuzzy Logic	robust and capable of handling data uncertainty	strict regulations that lack flexibility
Hough Transform	Identifies shape similarity with ease	Only spherical signal forms are detected.
Seed Based Region Growing Algorithms	Detect edges	User-defined parameters govern edge detection.
K-Means Clustering	Threshold values detected automatically	Cannot separate overlapping cells
Genetic Algorithms	Effectively searching for a suitable solutions	Slow
Active Contours	Boundaries are plainly discernible.	Energy conservation takes time.

2. Classification		
Support Vector Machines	Overfitting is unlikely to occur, and decision trees are easy to maintain.	It is challenging to get optical parameters for nonlinear data, and the training process is time-consuming.
K-Nearest Neighbour	sturdy, quick, and noise-tolerant	Attributes increases, the complexity also climbs, and it's not always true that instances sharing the same features are identical.
Bayesian Networks	It is simple to grasp and relies on statistical inference.	assumes that numerical attributes have a normal distribution and that they are statistically independent.
Genetic Algorithms	Look for a good solution that is optimized.	It is typically not the most efficient because it finds local optima.
Artificial Neural Networks	Resilient to noise, capable of utilizing multiple instances for classification.	Overfitting when dealing with sophisticated algorithms and numerous attributes

2.3. SUMMARY

The prediction of cervical cancer, feature extraction and selection, early-stage diagnosis, and classification techniques were all covered in detail, according to a summary. A thorough examination is carried out to determine which algorithm will work best in the future. By utilizing our past expertise in these techniques, we can concentrate on creating sophisticated algorithms for medical picture processing. The majority of the algorithms covered here have specific shortcomings, such as long calculation durations, computational complexity, segmentation faults, low accuracy, and the requirement for initialization. The primary goal of this work is to address these issues and provide a robust, efficient, quick, and low-complexity algorithm for segmenting cervical cancer images. Numerous studies are continuously being conducted since early Pap smear image screening is crucial for detecting cervical cancer. The qualities and attributes of the current approaches are primarily to blame for these breakthroughs. The cervical cancer diagnosis is fully summarized in this literature.

2.4. RESEARCH GAP

- Many studies focus on isolated data sources, such as Pap smear images or clinical data, without integrating multiple types of data (e.g., genetic, histological, and demographic data) for a more comprehensive diagnosis.

- There is limited research on the practical challenges and solutions for implementing machine learning models in clinical practice, such as integration with existing workflows and acceptance by healthcare providers.
- Emerging techniques, such as advanced deep learning architectures and hybrid models, are not extensively explored in the context of cervical cancer detection

CHAPTER – 3: PROGNOSIS OF CERVICAL CANCER DISEASE BY APPLYING MACHINE LEARNING TECHNIQUES

Every year, millions of women are impacted by cervical cancer, making it a serious worldwide health concern. Reducing death rates requires early detection. This chapter examines machine learning (ML) methods for cervical cancer detection and prediction. Using the UCI cervical cancer dataset, which includes the medical records of 858 individuals with 36 risk factors, six machine learning classifiers—Artificial Neural Network (ANN), Bayesian Network, Support Vector Machine (SVM), Random Tree, Logistic Regression, and XGBoost—were evaluated. Feature selection methods like Relief Rank, Wrapper Method, and LASSO Regression were applied to enhance model performance. The XGBoost classifier achieved the highest accuracy of 94.94% while using the complete feature set. The study demonstrates how machine learning may be used to develop reliable decision-support tools for cervical cancer prognostic prediction.

3.1. INTRODUCTION

Cervical cancer, mostly caused by persistent infection with high-risk strains of the human papillomavirus (HPV), is ace of the leading causes of cancer-related deaths among women worldwide. Even while HPV vaccinations and screening initiatives are successful in high-income nations, there are still major obstacles in low-resource environments. Early on, the disease is asymptomatic, which makes prompt detection more difficult and highlights the need for novel diagnostic techniques.

In the healthcare industry, machine learning has become a potent tool that makes it possible to analyze large, complicated information and extract predictive characteristics. This chapter examines how well ML classifiers use clinical, lifestyle, and demographic characteristics to predict cervical cancer.

3.2. RELATED WORK

Numerous studies have leveraged ML for cervical cancer prediction. For instance, Sunny Sharma used decision trees to classify cancer stages, aiding oncologists in treatment planning. Studies by S. Geeitha and M. Thangamani demonstrated the superior performance of SVM combined with Synthetic Minority Over - sampling Technique (SMOTE) for imbalanced datasets. Similarly, Zaridah S explored the use of HPV vaccination and screening programs to mitigate cervical cancer risks in Malaysia.

However, gaps remain in optimizing feature selection and exploring ensemble classifiers like XGBoost for improved accuracy. This study addresses these gaps by comparing the performance of multiple classifiers and incorporating advanced feature selection techniques.

3.3. METHODOLOGY

3.3.1. Description of the Dataset

The UCI cervical cancer dataset was utilized, comprising 858 samples with 36 attributes, including demographic data, sexual history, and medical test results. Target variables included outcomes from four specific medical tests: Schiller, Hinselmann, Cytology, and Biopsy. 30% of the dataset used for testing, while 70% used for training.

3.3.2. Feature Selection Techniques

To enhance model performance, three feature selection methods were employed:

- **Relief Rank:** Prioritizes features based on their relevance to the target variable.
- **Wrapper Method:** Iteratively selects subsets of features to optimize model performance.
- **LASSO Regression:** Reduces dimensionality by applying an L1 penalty to regression coefficients.

3.3.3. Classification Algorithms

Six classifiers were evaluated:

1. **Artificial Neural Network (ANN):** A supervised learning algorithm simulating interconnected neural nodes.
2. **Bayesian Network:** A probabilistic graphical model capturing dependencies between variables.

3. **Support Vector Machine (SVM):** Constructs hyperplanes to classify data points in high-dimensional spaces.
4. **Random Tree:** Builds multiple decision trees and aggregates their predictions.
5. **Logistic Regression:** Predicts binary outcomes based on input features.
6. **XGBoost:** An ensemble learning method optimizing decision trees for performance.

3.3.4. Performance Metrics

Model performance was evaluated using the following metrics:

- **Accuracy:** The percentage of cases that are accurately classified.
- **Precision:** The proportion of accurate positive forecasts to all positive forecasts.
- **Recall:** The ratio of genuine positive forecasts to actual positives is known as recall (sensitivity).
- **F1 – Score:** The F1-score is the harmonic mean of recall and precision.
- **AUC:** The model's capacity to differentiate between classes is gauged by the Area Under the Curve (AUC).

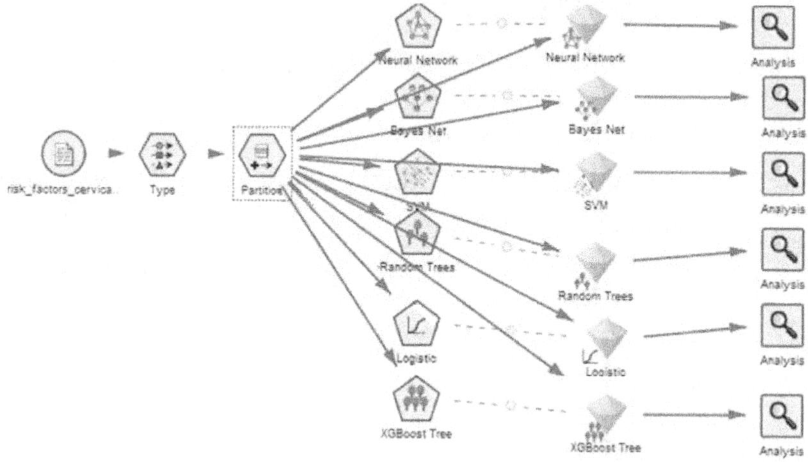

Figure 3.1 Cervical Cancer Prediction Model Using IBM SPSS

3.4. RESULTS

3.4.1. Classifier Performance Without Feature Selection

Using all dataset features, the XGBoost classifier achieved the highest accuracy of 94.94%, with a precision of 95.12%, recall of 99.69%, and an F1-score of 97.36%. ANN also performed well, achieving an accuracy of 92.33%. In contrast, SVM demonstrated the lowest accuracy at 49.90%.

Table 3.1 Classifier Performance Without Feature Selection

	Precision	Recall	F-Measure	AUC	GINI Coefficient	Accuracy
ANN	92.76%	99.42%	95.97%	64.50%	0.29	92.33%
Bayes Net	93.85%	98.61%	96.17%	80.60%	0.61	64.88%
SVM	63.47%	59.52%	63.75%	78.10%	0.56	49.90%
Random Tree	95.31%	96%	95.46%	86.40%	0.727	91.81%
Logistic	95.01%	98.88%	96.91%	93.00%	0.86	80.06%
XG Boost Tree	95.12%	99.69%	97.36%	85.10%	0.702	94.94%

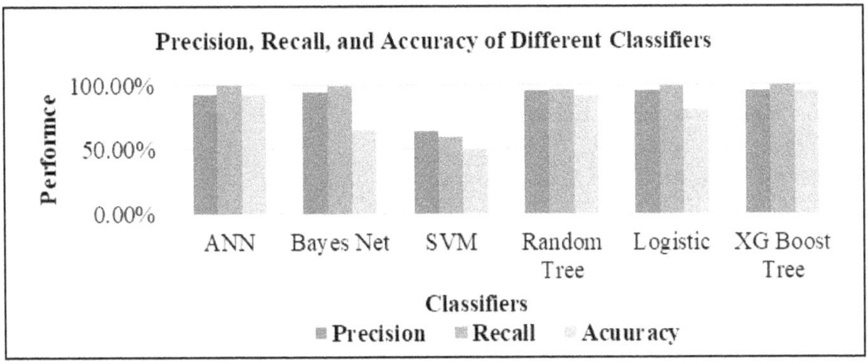

Figure 3.2 Comparison of all classifier's precision, recall, and accuracy without feature selections

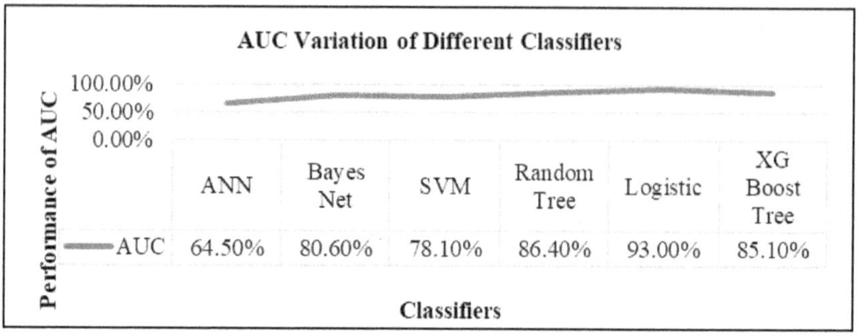

Figure 3.3 All Classifiers' Area Under Curve (AUC) Performance Without Feature Selections

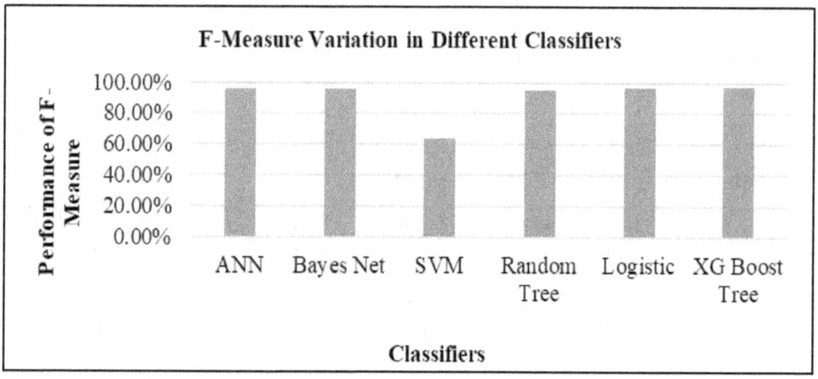

Figure 3.4 All Classifiers' F-Measures Perform Without Feature Selections

3.4.2. Impact of Feature Selection

Relief Rank

The Random Tree classifier achieved the highest accuracy (92.47%) with Relief Rank-selected features. This approach reduced dimensionality while maintaining classifier performance.

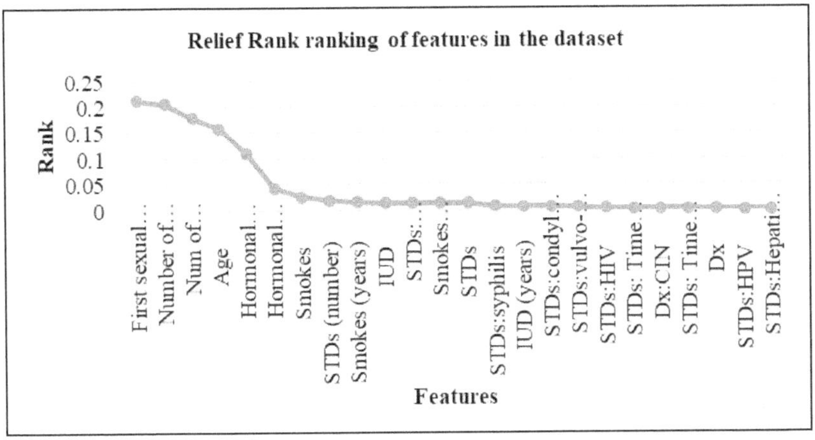

Figure 3.5 Importance of Dataset Features Using Relief Rank Algorithm

Table 3.2 Classifier performance after Relief Rank Algorithm

	Precision	Recall	F-Measure	AUC	GINI Coefficient	Accuracy
ANN	89.72%	100.00%	94.58%	73.90%	0.478	89.75%
Bayes Net	92.15%	98.73%	95.33%	64.10%	0.282	77.20%
SVM	93.88%	95.60%	94.73%	79.60%	0.592	78.43%
Random Tree	96.09%	96%	95.93%	79.80%	0.596	92.47%
Logistic	89.61%	100.00%	94.52%	74.20%	0.485	77.59%
XG Boost Tree	91.42%	100%	95.51%	80.50%	0.61	91.47%

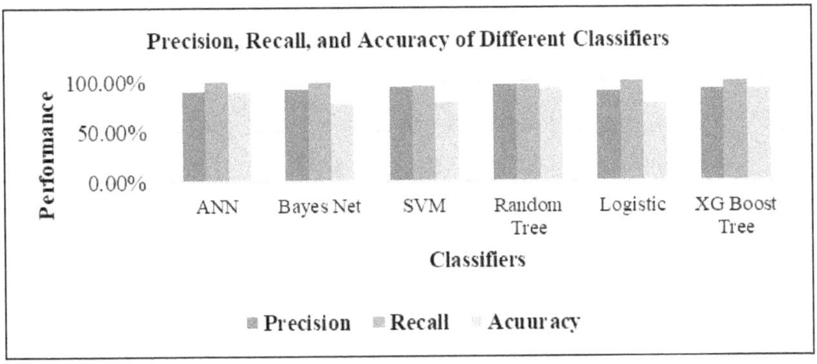

Figure 3.6 Classifier performance metrics after Relief Rank feature selection

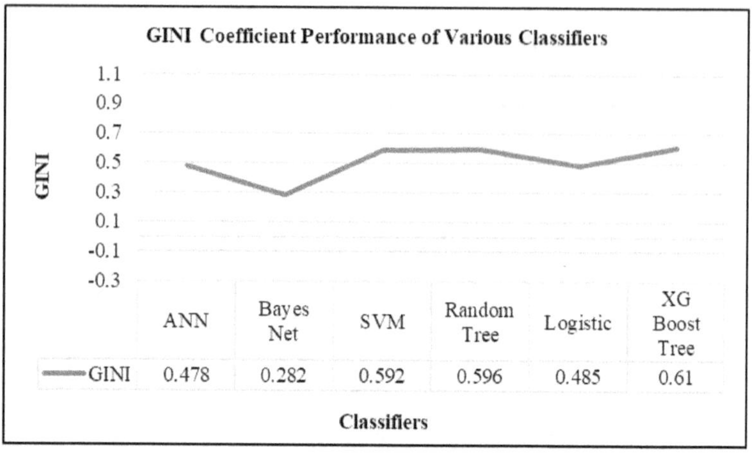

Figure 3.7 After the Relief Rank Algorithm performance of Gini Index of all Classifiers

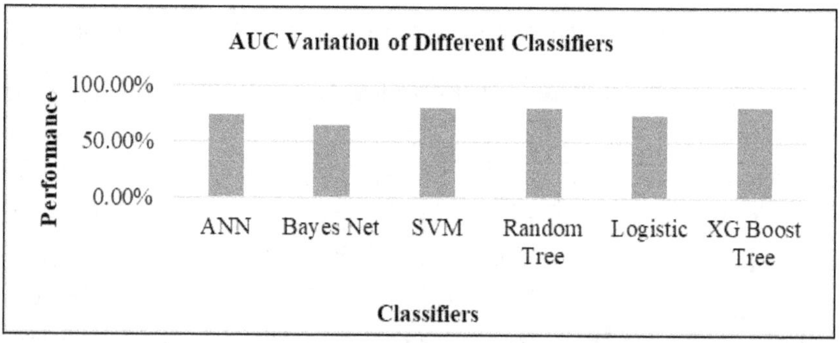

Figure 3.8 All Classifiers' Area Under Curve (AUC) Performance after Relief Rank Algorithm

Wrapper Method

The ANN classifier performed best with Wrapper-selected features, achieving 93.24% accuracy. This method highlighted the importance of iterative feature subset selection in enhancing performance.

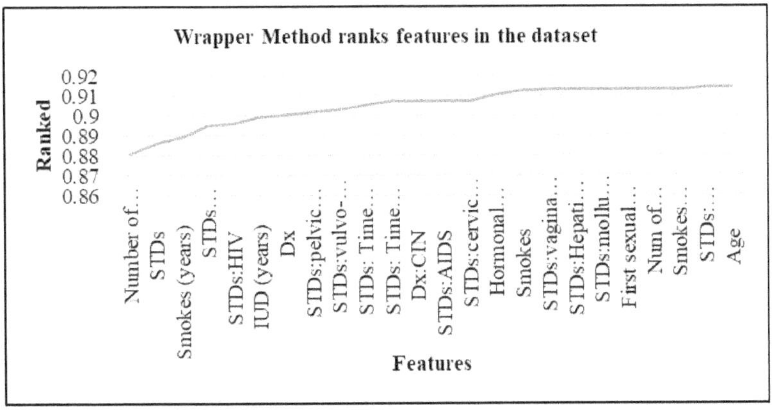

Figure 3.9 **Wrapper Forward Algorithm to Determine the Importance of Dataset Features**

Table 3.3 **Performance of Classifiers After Wrapper Forward Feature Selection**

	Precision	Recall	F-Measure	AUC	GINI Coefficient	Accuracy
ANN	93.43%	99.68%	96.45%	65.60%	0.31	93.24%
Bayes Net	93.92%	98.87%	96.33%	76.30%	0.53	75.63%
SVM	91.94%	98.04%	94.89%	74.80%	0.497	79.22%
Random Tree	94.77%	83%	88.45%	78.50%	0.57	80.28%
Logistic	92.20%	99.63%	95.77%	80.40%	0.609	79.66%
XG Boost Tree	91.69%	99.68%	95.52%	72.80%	0.457	91.43%

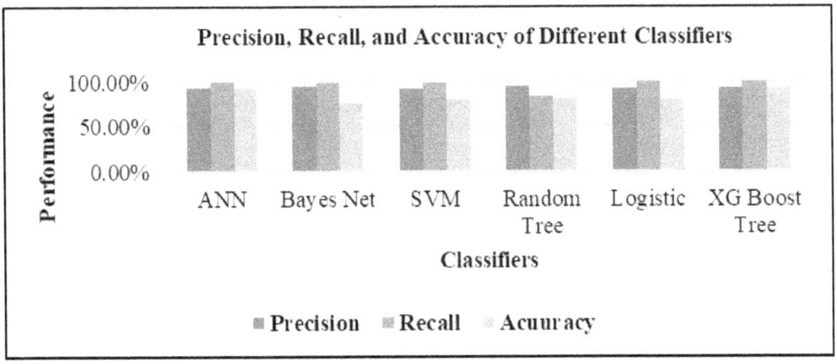

Figure 3.10 **Comparison of all classifiers precision, recall, and accuracy after wrapper forward feature selection**

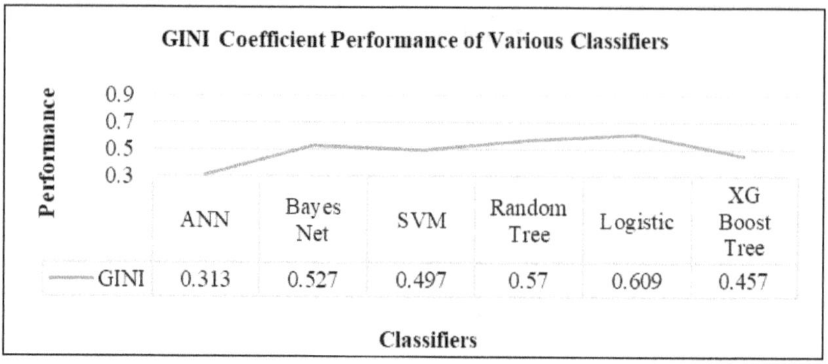

Figure 3.11 Gini Index Performance After Wrapper Forward Feature Selection

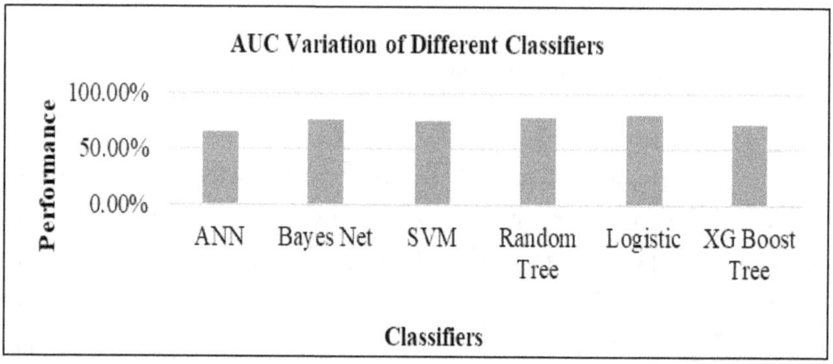

Figure 3.12 All Classifiers' Area Under Curve (AUC) Performance after Wrapper Forward Feature Selection

LASSO Regression

SVM demonstrated the highest accuracy (92.12%) with LASSO-selected features, emphasizing the utility of L1 regularization for feature reduction.

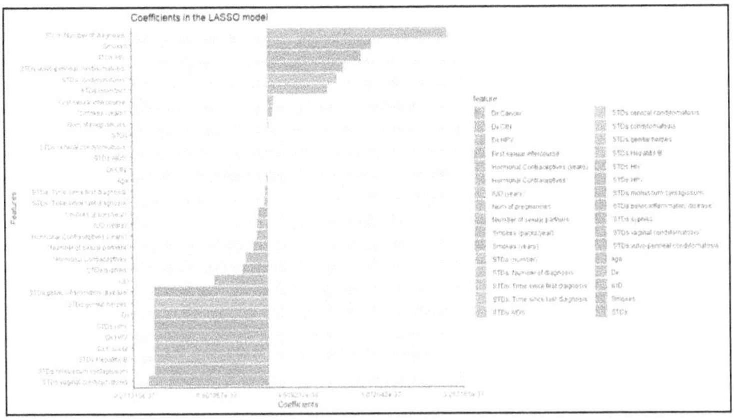

Figure 3.13 Lasso Regression Algorithm to Determine Dataset Feature Importance

Table 3.4 After Lasso Feature Selection, Classifier Performance

	Precision	Recall	F-Measure	AUC	GINI Coefficient	Accuracy
ANN	91.96%	100.00%	95.18%	58.70%	0.175	91.99%
Bayes Net	89.99%	99.62%	94.55%	58.70%	0.174	77.36%
SVM	92.07%	100.00%	95.87%	52.10%	0.043	92.12
Random Tree	91.56%	98%	94.59%	51.50%	0.03	89.80%
Logistic	88.88%	86.55%	87.80%	63.90%	0.278	78.11%
XG Boost Tree	89.45%	100%	94.29%	64.00%	0.28	89.20%

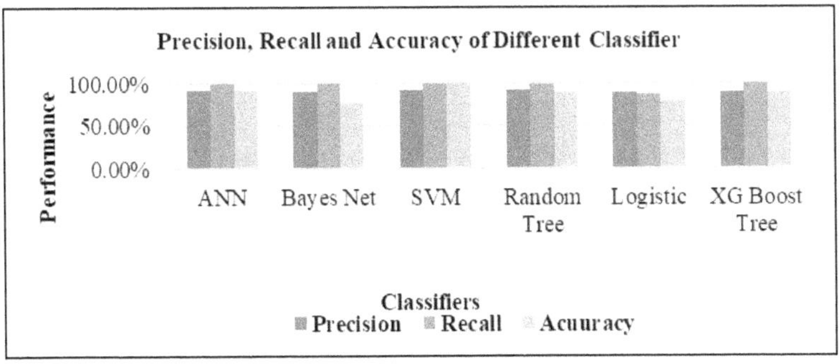

Figure 3.14 Comparison of all Classifiers' Precision, Recall, and Accuracy after Lasso Feature Selection

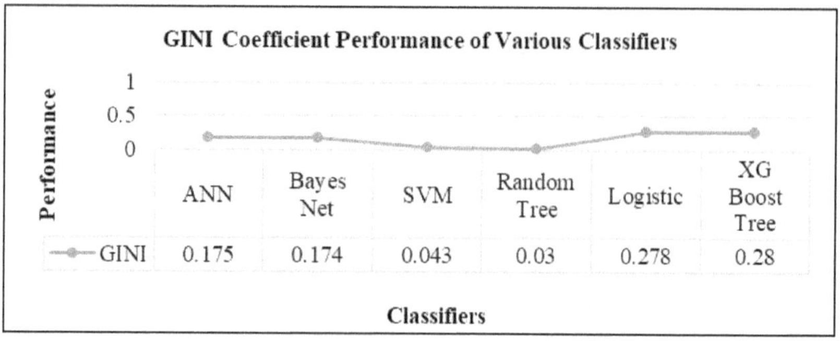

Figure 3.15 Gini Index Performance After Lasso Feature Selection

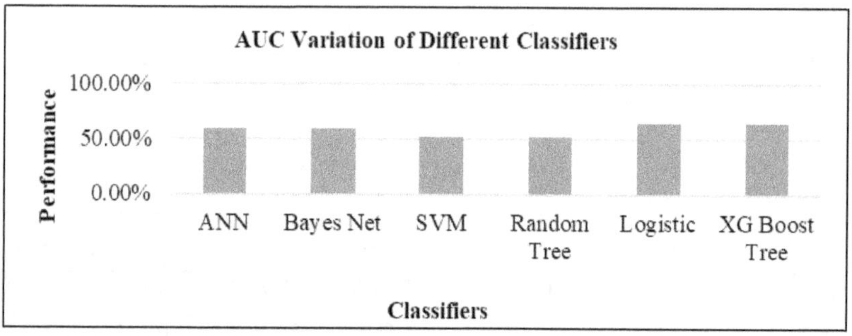

Figure 3.16 AUC Performance After Lasso Feature Selection

3.4.3. Comparative Analysis

Table 3.5 Classifier Performance in Various Model

	Full Features	Relief Rank	Wrapper FS	LASSO FS
ANN	92.33%	89.75%	93.24%	91.99%
Bayes Net	64.88%	77.20%	75.63%	77.36%
SVM	49.90%	78.43%	79.22%	92.12%
Random Tree	91.81%	92.47%	80.28%	89.80%
Logistic	80.06%	77.59%	79.66%	78.11%
XG Boost Tree	94.94%	91.47%	91.43%	89.20%

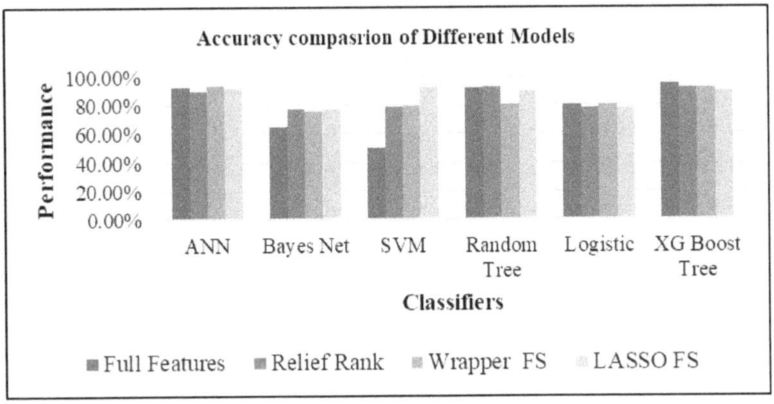

Figure 3.17 Comparison of all Classifier Models

3.5. DISCUSSION

3.5.1. Key Findings

- The XGBoost classifier consistently demonstrated superior performance, achieving the highest accuracy with the full feature set.
- Feature selection methods significantly improved classifier performance by reducing noise and enhancing relevant attributes.
- ANN and SVM performed well when combined with Wrapper and LASSO methods, respectively.

3.5.2. Limitations

- The dataset's size and imbalance posed challenges for model generalization.
- Some classifiers, such as BayesNet, struggled with high-dimensional data.

3.5.3. Real-World Implications

The proposed ML models offer a promising approach for early cervical cancer detection. Integrating such systems into clinical workflows could enhance diagnostic accuracy and reduce healthcare burdens.

3.6. CONCLUSION

This study highlights the potential of ML techniques in predicting cervical cancer. XGBoost emerged as the most effective classifier, achieving 94.94% accuracy with the complete feature set. Feature selection methods further improved model performance, underscoring their importance in handling high-dimensional datasets. Future research should focus on expanding datasets, exploring deep learning approaches, and incorporating diverse patient attributes to enhance model robustness and applicability.

CHAPTER - 4: BUILDING A DEEP LEARNING MODEL USING COLPOSCOPY IMAGES TO CLASSIFY CERVIX TYPES

4.1. INTRODUCTION

The creation and assessment of a deep learning model for cervix type classification using colposcopy pictures is presented in this chapter. The dataset included 200 photos that were annotated by medical experts and divided into three categories (Type 1, Type 2, and Type 3). Three cutting-edge deep learning architectures were used: VGG19, Inception v3, and ResNet50, all of which used pre-trained ImageNet weights. The models were trained, validated, and tested using standard evaluation metrics such as F1-score, accuracy, precision, and recall. Overall accuracy of 83.5% was achieved across all cervix types. Sensitivity ranged from 75.8% to 87.0%, while specificity varied between 84.7% and 93.0%. The proposed approach demonstrates potential for advancing automated cervix classification systems, aiding in early cervical cancer detection, and enhancing clinical decision-making.

4.2. RESEARCH GAP

Despite advancements in ML and DL, limited research has concentrating on leveraging feature fusion techniques to combine the strengths of multiple pre-trained models for cervical cancer detection. Addressing this gap could improve diagnostic accuracy and applicability in resource-limited settings.

4.3. OBJECTIVES

This study's main goal is to use characteristics taken from the Inception v3, VGG19, and ResNet50 models to categorize cervical cancer colposcopy images into Type 1, Type 2, and Type 3 groups. The research aims to answer the question: *Can the fusion of features from multiple pre-trained CNN models improve classification accuracy compared to individual models?*

4.4. METHODOLOGY

4.4.1. Data Acquisition

High-resolution colposcopy images were collected from hospital records, encompassing diverse cervical conditions. The dataset included 80 Type_1, 38 Type_2, and 38 Type_3 images, annotated by medical experts.

4.4.2. Preprocessing

Standard preprocessing steps included:

- **Resizing:** Images resized to 224×224 pixels.
- **Normalization:** Pixel values standardized to a range of 0 to 1.
- **Augmentation:** Techniques like rotation and flipping applied to enhance data diversity and reduce overfitting.

4.4.3. Feature Extraction

The last layers of the previously trained models were used to extract features:

- **Inception v3:** Features from the final pooling layer.
- **VGG19:** Features from fully connected layers.
- **ResNet50:** Features from residual blocks. The extracted features were concatenated to form a composite feature vector.

4.4.4. Model Architecture

The proposed architecture involved:

1. **Feature Fusion:** Combining features from Inception v3, VGG19, and ResNet50.
2. **Dimensionality Reduction:** Using Principal Component Analysis (PCA) to reduce the feature vector size.
3. **Classification:** Applying ML classifiers, including SVM, random forest, and neural networks, to the reduced feature vector.

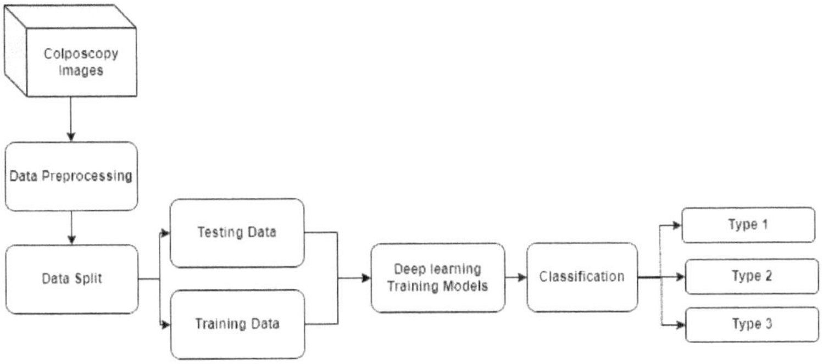

Figure 4.1 Block Diagram for the Suggested Approach

4.4.5. Parameters

The parameters for the proposed model include hyperparameters for both the feature extraction and classification stages. These parameters were optimized through cross-validation to achieve the best performance.

- Inception v3:
    - Input size: 224x224 pixels
    - Feature layer: Final pooling layer
    - Pre-trained weights: ImageNet
- VGG19:
    - Input size: 224x224 pixels
    - Feature layer: Fully connected layer
    - Pre-trained weights: ImageNet
- ResNet50:
    - Input size: 224x224 pixels
    - Feature layer: Residual block outputs
    - Pre-trained weights: ImageNet
- Feature Fusion:
    - Method: Concatenation
    - Dimensionality reduction: PCA
    - Number of components: Determined through cross-validation

- Classifiers:
  - SVM:
    - Kernel: Radial Basis Function (RBF)
    - C (regularization parameter): Tuned via grid search
    - Gamma: Tuned via grid search
  - Random Forest:
    - Number of trees: 100
    - Max depth: Tuned via cross-validation
  - Neural Network:
    - Architecture: Multi-layer perceptron
    - Number of layers: Tuned via cross-validation
    - Learning scale: 0.001
    - Bunch size: 32
    - Epochs: 50

4.5. RESULTS AND DISCUSSION

4.5.1. Model Performance

Performance metrics for each model and cervix type are summarized in Table 4.1.

Table 4.1 Performance metrics for each model and cervix type

Models	**Cervix_Type**	**Precision**	**Recall**	**F1-Score**
VGG19	Type_1	0.75	0.82	0.78
	Type_2	0.68	0.75	0.71
	Type_3	0.72	0.68	0.7
Inception v3	Type_1	0.82	0.79	0.8
	Type_2	0.74	0.8	0.77
	Type_3	0.69	0.65	0.67
ResNet50	Type_1	0.79	0.75	0.77
	Type_2	0.72	0.78	0.75
	Type_3	0.68	0.62	0.65

4.5.2. Transfer Learning Impact

Using pre-trained weights significantly enhanced performance on the small dataset. Inception v3 achieved the highest overall accuracy of 86%, highlighting the efficacy of transfer learning and feature fusion.

4.5.3. Real-world Applicability

The proposed model demonstrated robust specificity (84.7% to 93.0%) and sensitivity (75.8% to 87.0%), underscoring its potential for real-world deployment in cervical cancer screening programs.

4.6. CONCLUSION

This study introduces a novel feature fusion approach using Inception v3, VGG19, and ResNet50 models to classify cervical cancer colposcopy images. The results highlight the advantages of combining multiple pre-trained models to improve diagnostic accuracy. Future work should explore the integration of larger and more diverse datasets, refined architectures, and hybrid DL-ML models to further enhance classification performance.

CHAPTER - 5: CERVICAL CANCER PREDICTION USING MACHINE LEARNING TECHNIQUES

Medical care is frequently more expensive than preventative measures. Diseases like cervical cancer that are detected early have a far higher chance of being successfully treated, which improves survival rates and lowers mortality. Using information from the UCI cervical cancer risk factor dataset, a machine learning-based framework for cervical cancer prediction is presented in this chapter. To increase sensitivity and precision, the method incorporates Decision Tree, Random Forest, SMOTE to solve dataset imbalance and maximize model performance. Results indicate that major diagnostic techniques, such as the Schiller, Hinselmann, Cytology, and Biopsy tests, have improved sensitivity, accuracy, and ROC AUC for cervical cancer prediction.

5.1. INTRODUCTION

Cervical cancer is the fourth most common disease in women worldwide, and risk factors include age, hormonal contraception, and HPV infection. According to the World Health Organization (WHO), HPV vaccination and early screening tests can help prevent cervical cancer. By using machine learning (ML) to increase the accuracy and efficacy of early cervical cancer diagnosis, patient outcomes can be improved.

Developing a machine learning framework that integrates Decision Tree, Random Forest, and Logistic Regression classifiers is the aim of this study. The technique addresses problems with dataset imbalance and dimensionality while enhancing classification using SMOTE and PCA techniques.

5.2. RELATED WORK

Research emphasizes the importance of early cervical cancer detection to reduce mortality. Past studies have explored diverse ML techniques for cervical cancer prediction:

- **Abdoh et al.** applied Random Forest with SMOTE to address dataset imbalance, achieving improved classification accuracy.

- **Tanimu et al.** compared XGBoost, Random Forest, and SVM classifiers for cervical cancer classification, demonstrating the effectiveness of ensemble methods.
- **Arora et al.** used gene sequence datasets to develop scalable cervical cancer prediction models with high sensitivity.

These studies highlight the need for integrating advanced techniques like SMOTE and PCA to handle dataset challenges and enhance model performance.

5.3. RESEARCH METHODOLOGY

5.3.1. Dataset Description

The UCI cervical cancer dataset contains 858 samples with 32 attributes, covering demographic, medical, and lifestyle risk factors. Four diagnostic tests (Schiller, Hinselmann, Cytology, and Biopsy) serve as target variables.

5.3.2. Data Preprocessing

- **Handling Missing Values:** Missing values were imputed using mean-based and decision-tree-based approaches.
- **Outlier Detection:** Extreme values were identified and managed to improve data quality.
- **Feature Scaling:** Attributes were normalized for better model performance.

5.3.3. Techniques

- **Synthetic Minority Oversampling Technique (SMOTE):** Increased the minority class population to balance the dataset.
- **Principal Component Analysis (PCA):** Reduced dimensionality while retaining critical information.
- **Cross-Validation:** Applied tenfold stratified cross-validation to ensure robust performance evaluation.

5.3.4. Classification Algorithms

- **Logistic Regression:** Used for binary outcome prediction based on independent variables.
- **Decision Tree:** A hierarchical model based on feature splits.
- **Random Forest:** An ensemble of decision trees for improved accuracy and reduced overfitting.
- **Voting Classifier:** Combined predictions from the three classifiers for final output.

5.4. EXPERIMENTAL RESULTS

5.4.1. Hinselmann Test

The model achieved 97.15% accuracy after applying SMOTE and PCA, with sensitivity increasing from 50.68% to 97.87%. The ROC AUC improved from 65.48% to 97.97%.

5.4.2. Schiller Test

Accuracy improved from 89.91% to 96.17% after SMOTE application, with sensitivity increasing by 35.65%. The ROC AUC reached 99.8% with SMOTE and PCA.

5.4.3. Cytology Test

The Cytology model achieved an accuracy of 94.05% with SMOTE and PCA, showing significant improvements in sensitivity (92.98%) and ROC AUC (94.25%).

5.4.4. Biopsy Test

For Biopsy, the final model attained an accuracy of 98.78%, with sensitivity and ROC AUC increasing to 98.01% and 99.57%, respectively.

Table 5.1 Performance Summary

Metric	Hinselmann	Schiller	Cytology	Biopsy
Accuracy (%)	97.15	96.17	94.05	98.78
Sensitivity (%)	97.87	93.47	92.98	98.01
ROC AUC (%)	97.97	99.8	94.25	99.57

5.5. DISCUSSION

Key Findings

- The integration of SMOTE and PCA significantly enhanced sensitivity and accuracy for all diagnostic tests.
- The Voting Classifier demonstrated superior performance compared to individual classifiers, leveraging their combined strengths.
- The approach effectively addressed dataset imbalance, a common challenge in medical data analysis.

Limitations

- The dataset's size limited generalizability. Larger datasets are needed for broader applicability.
- The model's performance may vary with additional features or alternative classification techniques.

5.6. CONCLUSION

This study highlights the potential of machine learning techniques in cervical cancer prediction. By combining SMOTE, PCA, and ensemble classifiers, the framework achieved high sensitivity and accuracy across diagnostic tests. These findings can inform clinical decision-making, enabling early detection and treatment of cervical cancer.

CHAPTER - 6: INNOVATIVE MACHINE LEARNING METHODS FOR CERVICAL CANCER PREDICTION

Preventative methods are often less expensive than medical procedures. Early detection of diseases like cervical cancer can significantly improve recovery rates and reduce mortality. The primary objective of this chapter is to develop a machine learning system that can accurately and sensitively predict cervical cancer. By integrating Decision Tree, Random Forest, and Logistic Regression classifiers into a voting mechanism, the proposed method addresses dataset imbalance by using Synthetic Minority Oversampling Technique (SMOTE) and Principal Component Analysis (PCA) to minimize dimensionality. The framework employs stratified 10-fold cross-validation to ensure a reliable assessment. The findings demonstrate that the proposed model improves prediction accuracy, sensitivity, and ROC-AUC for all significant diagnostic methods, such as the Hinselmann, Cytology, Schiller, and Biopsy tests. This paper demonstrates the value of ensemble techniques in combination with SMOTE and PCA for cervical cancer prediction.

6.1. INTRODUCTION

Cervical cancer is ace of the leading reasons of cancer related death for women globally. Chronic high-risk human papillomavirus (HPV) infection is often the cause of this fourth most common cancer in women. Age, the use of hormonal contraception and the number of sexual partners are risk factors for cervical cancer. Effective screening techniques and immunization programs enable early diagnosis, which dramatically lowers mortality and increases recovery rates.

Machine learning (ML) offers advanced tools for analyzing complex datasets and extracting meaningful patterns. This study explores ML techniques to improve cervical cancer prediction using data from the UCI dataset. The approach employs ensemble methods to combine the strengths of Logistic Regression, Decision Tree, and Random Forest classifiers, addressing the challenges of dataset imbalance and dimensionality.

6.2. RELATED WORK

Past research highlights the importance of early detection for reducing cervical cancer fatalities. Studies have explored various ML models and techniques:

- Abdoh et al. demonstrated the efficacy of Random Forest classifiers combined with SMOTE for improving sensitivity and specificity in cervical cancer prediction.
- Wu and Zhou analyzed the influence of risk factors, such as the number of sexual partners and age at first sexual intercourse, using SVM-based approaches.
- Fernandes et al. introduced artificial neural networks for cervical cancer classification, emphasizing the role of feature reduction techniques.

These studies underscore the need for effective handling of imbalanced datasets and dimensionality reduction to improve prediction accuracy.

6.3. METHODOLOGY

6.3.1. Dataset Description

The UCI cervical cancer dataset consists of 858 samples and 32 attributes, including demographic, behavioral, and medical risk factors. The target variables represent diagnostic outcomes from four screening tests: Hinselmann, Cytology, Schiller, and Biopsy.

6.3.2. Data Preprocessing

- **Handling Missing Values:** Imputed using mean-based and decision-tree-based methods.
- **Feature Scaling:** Normalized feature values to ensure uniformity.
- **Outlier Detection:** Identified and managed anomalies to improve data quality.

6.3.3. Techniques

- **SMOTE:** Addressed class imbalance by synthesizing additional samples for minority classes.
- **PCA:** Reduced dimensionality by transforming data into principal components while retaining critical information.

- **Cross-Validation:** Used stratified 10-fold cross-validation to ensure reliable model evaluation.

6.3.4. Classification Algorithms

1. **Logistic Regression (LR):** Predicts binary outcomes based on input features.
2. **Decision Tree (DT):** Classifies data through hierarchical splits.
3. **Random Forest (RF):** Combines multiple decision trees to enhance accuracy and reduce overfitting.
4. **Voting Classifier:** Integrates predictions from LR, DT, and RF to improve performance.

6.4. RESULTS

6.4.1. Hinselmann Test

- Accuracy improved from 94.32% to 96.77% after applying SMOTE and PCA.
- Sensitivity increased from 63% to 96.98%, and ROC-AUC rose to 98.21%.

Table 6.1 Predictive Model Assessment for the Hinselmann Target Variable

Metric	Before applying SMOTE	After applying SMOTE
Accuracy (%)	94.32	96.77
Sensitivity (%)	63	96.98
ROC-AUC (%)	65.23	98.21

6.4.2. Schiller Test

- SMOTE improved accuracy from 89.36% to 95.1%.
- Sensitivity increased by 38.11%, and ROC-AUC reached 91.49%.

Table 6.2 Predictive Model Assessment for the Schiller Variable

Metric	Before SMOTE	After SMOTE
Accuracy (%)	89.36	95.1
Sensitivity (%)	56.21	94.32
ROC-AUC (%)	67.5	91.49

6.4.3. Cytology Test

- The SMOTE-PCA model achieved 94.3% sensitivity and 94.23% F1-score.
- Accuracy dropped slightly from 94.77% to 92.23%, but sensitivity improved significantly.

Table 6.3 Predictive Model Assessment for the Cytology Variable

Metric	Before SMOTE	After SMOTE
Accuracy (%)	93.69	92.23
Sensitivity (%)	53.48	92.2
ROC-AUC (%)	61.22	75.56

6.4.4. Biopsy Test

- SMOTE-PCA model achieved the highest accuracy of 98.23%.
- ROC-AUC reached 99.87%, with sensitivity at 98.12%.

Table 6.4 Predictive Model Assessment for the Biopsy Variable

Metric	Before SMOTE	After SMOTE
Accuracy (%)	94.3	98.23
Sensitivity (%)	53.45	98.12
ROC-AUC (%)	65.98	99.87

6.5. DISCUSSION

Key Findings

- SMOTE effectively addressed class imbalance, significantly improving sensitivity and prediction accuracy.
- PCA reduced computational complexity without compromising model performance.
- The Voting Classifier outperformed individual classifiers by leveraging their combined strengths.

Limitations

- Dataset size limited generalizability: larger datasets are needed.
- Additional features could enhance model robustness and accuracy.

6.6. CONCLUSION

The study demonstrates the efficacy of ensemble methods combined with SMOTE and PCA for predicting cervical cancer. By addressing class imbalance and dimensionality, the proposed framework achieved high sensitivity, accuracy, and ROC-AUC across all diagnostic tests. These findings highlight the potential of ML techniques in enhancing early detection and improving patient outcomes.

CHAPTER – 7: A COMBINED FRAMEWORK FOR FEATURE EXTRACTION AND CLASSIFICATION

7.1. INTRODUCTION

We outline the methodology used in developing the ColpoClassifier, a hybrid framework for classifying cervigrams. Cervical cancer screening is a critical preventive measure, and accurate classification of cervigrams can significantly enhance early detection and treatment outcomes. This methodology's goal is to develop a reliable and effective procedure that correctly classifies cervigrams by utilizing machine learning algorithms and sophisticated image processing techniques.

A summary of the dataset, including the kinds and numbers of photos utilized, opens the chapter. After that, it goes through the data preparation procedures required to get the pictures ready for examination. A key part of our approach is feature extraction, and we outline the methods used, particularly the Gray-Level Co-occurrence Matrix (GLCM) and Histogram of Oriented Gradients (HOG). These qualities are necessary to capture the texture and intricate structural details of the images.

Following the feature extraction, we discuss the classification techniques utilized, including Support Vector Machines (SVM) and Random Forests. We describe how these classifiers are trained, validated, and combined in our hybrid framework to improve classification performance. Implementation details, such as the software and tools used, are also provided to offer a comprehensive understanding of the methodological framework.

Noise and inconsistencies can creep into the image during development. Over the last 40 to 50 years, various procedures have been created in image processing. The majority of techniques have been created to improve photos taken by military surveillance flights, satellites, and space probes. Because compatible computers, high-capacity memory devices, and programming possibilities are widely available, image processing systems are growing in popularity. To overcome these deficiencies and achieve data innovation, you need to experience different periods of preparation.

- Image preprocessing
- Image enhancement
- Image analysis
- Image segmentation

7.1.1. Image Pre-processing

Image pre-processing is a step in the early phases of the image processing chain. This is the fundamental level of picture editing where intensity images are used as both the input and the output. By eliminating undesired distortions or ornamental particular aspects that are essential for further processing, Image preparation extends the nature of an image by reducing the amount of noise that appears in the image and emphasizing the features used as part of image sharing.

7.1.2. Image Enhancement

To improve an image's visual impact, image enhancement entails modifying the pixel brightness levels. This procedure consists of a number of actions intended to improve an image's visual appeal so that it is more enticing to human viewers. The pre-processed image contains noise that needs to be removed to further process the image. Image noise is most noticeable in low flag level image areas, such as in shadow areas or under bare images.

The goal of image enhancement is to emphasize certain characteristics of the image to be displayed (Jahne, 2005). The cabinet includes differences and edge enhancements, pseudo-blurring, noise filtering, sharpness, and magnification. Feature extraction, picture analysis, and display all benefit from image enhancement. The enhancement technique draws attention to particular standard elements of the image rather than changing the information's core data content. Intelligent, application-specific advanced algorithms are usually employed for enhancement. The main principle of the image filtering technique is to enhance, a hybrid median filtering method is implemented to improve the properties of the image and increase the brightness of the sample

7.1.3. Image Analysis

Richards and Richards (1999) suggested image analysis quantifies an image to represent the image. With the slightest problem, the project can read a food's label, line up the various pieces on a conveyor belt, measure its size, and place the platelets in a medical photo. Developed image analysis systems also measure and use quantitative data to arrive at a modern option, such as controlling a robotic arm to move a question for the detection or examining an airship with evidence from images. Image inspection methods require the extraction of specific features that guide the detection of a recognizable object.

7.1.4. Segmentation Approaches in Imaging

Segmentation is one of the most common steps in reducing images to data (John, 1999). Segmentation techniques have been used to limit the object from the scene to the target on which the estimates were made. The degree of this division depends on the problem under consideration, ie the division must be ended when the elements of the desired use are separated from the image and then the principle of possible communication is shared. Image segmentation algorithms depend on discontinuities or similarities in pixel estimation. The irregularity style divides the image based on sudden changes in intensity, edges, points, points, and lines in the image. In the same approach, a sequence of previous different criteria is used to divide the image into comparable areas according to the model set. Threshold, area growth, area segmentation, and aggregation are examples of similarity-based segmentation techniques.

7.1.5. Feature Extraction

The function extraction shows the important shape of the data in an example, so it is easy to organize the example with a formal system. An inventive method for lowering dimensionality in pattern recognition and image processing is feature extraction.

While condensing its representation is the main purpose of feature extraction. This is especially helpful when the algorithm's input data is too big to analyse efficiently and can contain redundant information, the input information is reduced to a set of image features.

Converting input information in the order of function is called feature extraction. Of course, with careful selection of individual features, the feature set will output the information available, and the goal is to accomplish the desired task with that small image input rather than full volume.

7.2. NEED FOR FEATURE EXTRACTION

If the algorithm information is too large to process and is suspect of redundancy, the information changes to a lower image feature set. Converting input information in the correct order is called a function extraction function. In this way, the science of distinguishing features enhances the reduction in information vector length by eliminating signal redundancy and compressing relevant data in a feature vector to completely reduce scaling. Magnetic resonance imaging is a graphic image in which specific data about the objects in the example are identified based on the type of defect. Thus, the MRI can be visualized with relevant features that can control the deformation. After extracting the relevant features, it makes sense to expand the method for recognizing the type of error detected. Various strategies have been used to separate features from images.

Among the often-employed methods are the following:

1. Spatial Characteristics
2. Histogram Features
3. Transformed Attributes
4. Boundary And Edge Descriptors
5. Color Metrics
6. Shape Descriptors
7. Texture Characteristics

7.2.1. Spatial Characteristics

Spatial properties of objects with a gray surface, amplitude, and spatial spread were described. One of an object's most essential and important characteristics is its capacity. The adaptive properties of the weights are reflected in the amplitude of X-rays, which makes it possible to distinguish between tissue and bone.

7.2.2. Histogram Features

The intensity values of an image's pixels are represented by its histogram. It shows how many pixels there are in the image at each intensity level. An image's histogram, which displays the distribution of pixels across grayscale values, is shown in Figure 4.1. 256

different intensity levels are conceivable in an 8-bit grayscale picture. A region with low contrast is shown by a narrow histogram. The mean, variance, standard deviation, energy, skewness, median, and kurtosis are typical histogram features.

7.2.3. Transformed Attributes

In most cases, the image conversion provides information about the frequency range. Image conversion functions are extracted using a regional filter. It is also known as a feature mask where the veil is slit or open. Boundaries and edges are usually detected using high-frequency components. The background can be identified with the aid of corner detection. When the input data comes from transformed coordinates, it is also crucial to extract the transformation functions.

7.2.4. Boundary and Edge Descriptors

One of the hardest challenges in image processing is edge detection, which is a major area of study. Images' edges are regions of high contrast in intensity, where a sudden change in intensity from one pixel to the next can cause discernible changes in the quality of the image. By removing unnecessary information while maintaining an image's key characteristics, effective edge detection drastically lowers the amount of data. An edge has no width at a given scale, although edges vary in scale, and a single edge may contain several edges. Accurately detecting edges in an image allows for the identification of every object and the simple measurement of its basic characteristics, including shape and perimeter.

7.2.5. Color Metrics

An object's color is a visual attribute that results from the light it emits, transmits, or reflects. The color signal is a mathematical extension of scalar and vector signals. The histogram of a picture can be used to extract color information. The color histogram's drawback is that it can be the same for two distinct objects that have the same color. The suggested color moments strategy is predicated on the mathematical idea that any color distribution can be expressed in order to lessen the quantization effects observed in color histograms.

7.2.6. Shape Descriptors

An object's physical composition and profile are referred to as its form. The main purposes of form characteristics are to measure dimensions, identify and match shapes, and recognize things. Moments, area, perimeter, and orientation are some of the attributes used in the shape feature extraction procedure. An object's external boundary determines its shape, which is different from the object's spatial qualities and other attributes like color, texture, and material composition.

7.2.7. Texture Characteristics

A recurring pattern or arrangement of structures with regular intervals is referred to as texture. It basically refers to an object's surface characteristics and appearance, which are defined by elements like size, shape, density, organization, and the ratio of its basic constituents. Texture feature extraction obtaining these properties. This extraction procedure is essential to many image processing applications, such as medical imaging, and remote sensing, because of the importance of texture information. Many of the feature extraction strategies used in this work center on transformation approaches.

7.2.8. Transform Methods

Fourier, Gabor, and wavelet transforms are examples of transform techniques that express an image in a coordinate system that is closely related to texture properties. The performance of Fourier transform algorithms is impacted by their spatial resolution restriction. Although gabor filters provide better spatial localization, their applicability is limited because natural textures rarely have a single filter resolution that can successfully isolate spatial components. These methods entail applying filters to original photos, then figuring out how much energy the altered images contain. They might not be appropriate for applications that concentrate on particular aspects of the input photos, though, as they frequently rely on the overall image processing. Wavelet transforms, on the other hand, offer a more suitable foundation for image processing according to its functional characteristics. The benefits of wavelet transform include:

- Energy compaction is the capacity to condense the majority of the signal's energy into a limited number of transformation coefficients.

- Another significant benefit is the capacity to efficiently record and depict both high-frequency transients (like image borders) and low-frequency elements (like image backgrounds).
- Another important advantage is that variable resolution decomposition with nearly uncorrelated coefficients can be achieved.
- Progressive transmission makes it possible to receive images with different quality levels.

7.2.9. Feature Selection

While several characteristics can be employed to characterize an image, feature selection plays a crucial role in many pattern recognition issues (Guyon and Elisseeff 2003). While several characteristics can be employed to characterize an image, feature selection plays a crucial role in many pattern recognition issues (Guyon and Elisseeff 2003). just a couple of them are productive and compelling in classifications. More features do not generally prompt a superior grouping execution, these lines include determination is typically performed to choose a smaller and applicable component subset considering the ultimate objective to diminish the dimensionality of feature space, which will in the end enhance the arrangement precision and reduces time utilization. Algorithms for feature selection are frequently employed in digital image machine learning jobs. Digital images are used for many things, such as segmentation, compression, improvement, and classification. Pixels with different intensities are placed in patterns to create each digital image.

Color, form, texture, and geometry are just a few examples of the unique characteristics that humans can use to identify and recognize various items. An object becomes identifiable when a new subset of it is shown because the brain compares it to the previously stored features in memory. Similar to this, a feature set comprising several distinguishing characteristics of the item of interest—whether it be digital photos or any quantifiable entity—is required for machine learning. After analysis, this collection of distinguishing characteristics is put via feature selection and classification procedures.

Figure 7.1 Feature Subset Selection shows the four main processes that make up the overall feature selection process.

- Evaluation of Feature Subsets
- Stopping Criterion
- Validation of Results

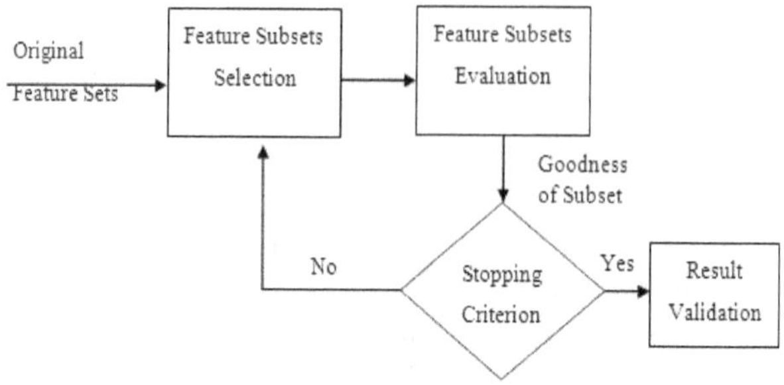

Figure 7.1 Feature Subset Selection Process

Feature Subset Selection is a heuristic hunt in which each state determines an applicant subset for assessment in the pursuit space. Two fundamental variables that impact the idea of the subset selection process are starting point and search organization. The search starting point chooses the course of the search. The accessible strategies are going ahead, going in reverse, hybrid method, weighting, and random methods. Using certain methods like random, exponential, or sequential search, the search strategy is in charge of the feature selection procedure.

In the evaluation phase of the functional subset, the newly created subset must be calculated using a specific evaluation criterion. Numerous assessment criteria have been suggested in the literature to assess the effectiveness of different subsets of identified traits.

Dependent criteria include predefined extraction algorithms for the feature selection. From the set of generated features, the one that offers the highest performance of the extraction algorithm is selected. This process ends when the termination criteria are met. This is not part of the feature selection process but involves a selection strategy that needs to be agreed upon by performing various experiments and correlating with previous stable results or screening against the effects of competing technologies through simulated data sets, real data sets, or both.

In light of various assessment measures, feature selection techniques can be characterized into three classes: embedded methods, filtering methods, and wrapper methods. Filter models use the qualities of feature information and are all the more computationally productive. Right off the bat, on account of embedded techniques for feature selection, such strategies are a piece of the indicators as on account of choice trees and neural systems. Filtering approaches, on the other hand, are based on rating the characteristics to determine their relevance from the chosen subset and function independently of the predictors. In filtering approaches, correlation, chi-square, and probability distribution are often used techniques for locating pertinent features. Wrapping around particular predictors to assess their performance is the third category, or "wrappers". This approach often divides the dataset into training and testing sets in order to assess the predictors' effectiveness.

7.3. CLASSIFICATION

One method that is frequently used in the diagnosis of diseases is classification. Predicting the target category for every item in the dataset with accuracy is its main goal. The classification has many uses in customer service, business modeling, marketing, credit analysis, biomedicine, and drug response modeling. When all is said and done, tendency or characterization falls into three major categories: centralized, unsupervised, and semi-structured.

7.3.1. Monitored Learning Strategies

A machine learning process used to extract skills from educational data. Mohari et al., (2012) Education data include the order of file creation. Each instance in supervised learning is represented as a pair consisting of the expected output (sometimes called the target or label) and an input object (often a feature vector).

In order to produce a derived function that can be used to produce predictions for fresh input instances, the supervised learning algorithm examines the training data. Ideally, consider an algorithm for effectively selecting class names for non-obvious events. For the learning algorithm to generalize well to unknown conditions, it must be well trained on the data.

7.3.2. Monitored Learning Techniques

Supervised learning encompasses all classification and regression procedures.

- Logistic Regression (LR)
- Decision Trees (DTs)
- Support Vector Machine (SVM)
- Naive Bayes (NBS)
- k-Nearest Neighbors (CNN)
- Linear Regression (LR)
- Random Forest (RF)
- Polynomial Regression (PR)

7.3.3. Unsupervised Learning

Unsupervised learning (Gramani, 2004) is the act of unlabeled information to separate specific input information. The process of machine learning is to predict the ability to visualize a hidden structure based on "unlabeled" ML information. Since the items given are not categorized for analysis, Unsupervised learning differs from supervised learning and reinforcement learning in that the correctness of the model produced by the algorithm is not assessed. Finding patterns or groupings in data without predetermined labels is the main goal of this method. Clustering, dimensionality reduction, and association analysis are methods used in unsupervised learning.

- Clustering
  - Mixture Models
  - K-Means
  - Exploring Hierarchical Clustering Algorithms,
- Understanding Anomaly Detection Algorithms
- Neural Networks(CNNs)
  - Hebbian Learning: Theory and Implementation
  - Understanding GANs: Techniques and Use Cases
- Exploring Diverse Learning Approaches
- EM Algorithm in Statistical Inference
- An Introduction to the Method of Moments
- Exploring Blind Source Separation Algorithms

- Feature Extraction via PCA,
- Independent Component Analysis(ICA),
- Techniques for Non-Negative Matrix Analysis,
- Exploring Singular Value Decomposition in Data Analysis

7.3.4. Semi-Supervised Learning

Semi-supervised learning (Zhou and Belkin, 2014) is a set of structured learning tasks and strategies that also use unlabeled information for preparation - usually a small amount of labeled information with a lot of unlabeled information. Semi-regulatory learning lies between learning without supervision (without marked start information) and monitored learning (with fully marked start information).

Many machine learning analysts have found that untagged information, when used as part of a relationship with a small amount of labeled information, can cause widespread changes in learning accuracy. To secure this information for a normal learning problem, a skilled human operator is required (e.g., transcribing an audio clip). The cost associated with the tagging method can make the fully tagged tutorial useless, although it is very cheap to buy untagged information. Semi-supervised learning can be very successful in these situations. This method is considered a model for human learning as well as a machine learning methodology.

The systematic approach taken to develop the ColpoClassifier, the rationale behind the chosen techniques, and the steps involved in training and validating the model. This foundation sets the stage for the subsequent presentation of results and their implications in the following chapter.

7.4. DATA GATHERING AND PREPARATION

Number of Images and Cases

The dataset consists of 1000 colposcopy images categorized into three types: Type 1, Type 2, and Type 3. These classifications will be provided by medical professionals based on clinical evaluations.

Images will undergo preprocessing to standardize size and quality, ensuring consistency for effective model training.

- **Type 1:** 570 Images
- **Type 2:** 230 images
- **Type 3:** 200 Images

Each type corresponds to distinct characteristics or conditions observed in cervigrams, crucial for classification tasks aimed at detecting abnormalities.

Types of Images

The images are categorized into three main types based on their visual characteristics and medical relevance:

Type 1: Images representing normal cervigrams.

Type 2: Images depicting cervigrams with mild abnormalities.

Type 3: Images showing cervigrams with severe abnormalities.

These categories enable the classification framework to differentiate between varying levels of cervical health conditions, aiding in early diagnosis and treatment planning.

Data Organization

Training and Testing Directories

The dataset is organized into separate directories for training and testing purposes, ensuring a structured approach to model development and evaluation:

Training Directory: Contains subdirectories for each type of image (type 1, type 2, type 3).

Testing Directory: Similar structure with separate subdirectories for each image type.

This organization facilitates systematic data handling and ensures that the models are trained and evaluated on distinct sets of data to assess generalizability and performance.

This hierarchical structure not only simplifies data access and management but also supports efficient batch processing and analysis during model training and testing phases.

7.5. DATA PRE-PROCESSING STEPS

Image Resizing and Normalization

Before feature extraction and model training, Preprocessing procedures are applied to the photos in order to standardize their format and enhance model performance.

- **Image Resizing:** To ensure consistency in input size across the dataset, all photos are shrunk to a standard size (e.g., 256x256 pixels).
- **Normalization:** Pixel intensity values are normalized to a common scale (e.g., [0, 1]) to mitigate variations in lighting conditions and enhance feature extraction accuracy.

These preprocessing steps contribute to reducing data variability and improving the robustness of the classification framework.

Handling Missing or Corrupt Images

To maintain data integrity and ensure the reliability of the classification models, specific measures are taken to address missing or corrupt images:

- **Missing Image Handling:** Images with missing data or file errors are flagged and excluded from further processing to prevent bias or errors in model training.
- **Corrupt Image Detection:** Automated checks are implemented to identify and remove images that exhibit file corruption or unreadable content, ensuring only valid data is used for analysis.

7.6. FEATURE EXTRACTION

In the Colpo Classifier framework, the GLCM and HOG are the two main feature extraction methods used to extract important features from cervigram pictures.

Gray-Level Co-occurrence Matrix (GLCM)

Explanation of GLCM

A texture analysis method called the Gray-Level Co-occurrence Matrix (GLCM) quantifies the spatial correlations between pixel pairs at predetermined angles and distances inside an image. It measures how often pairs of pixel intensities occur together at specified offsets.

Computation of Co-occurrence Matrix

- The collection of potential pixel values is represented by the rows and columns, which have N X N (N = Number of Gray values).
- It is calculated using two factors.
- d (Pixel number, such as 1, 2,...) indicates the relative distance between the pair of pixels.
- θ (Rotational angle and relative orientation, such as 0°, 45°, 90°, 135°, etc.)

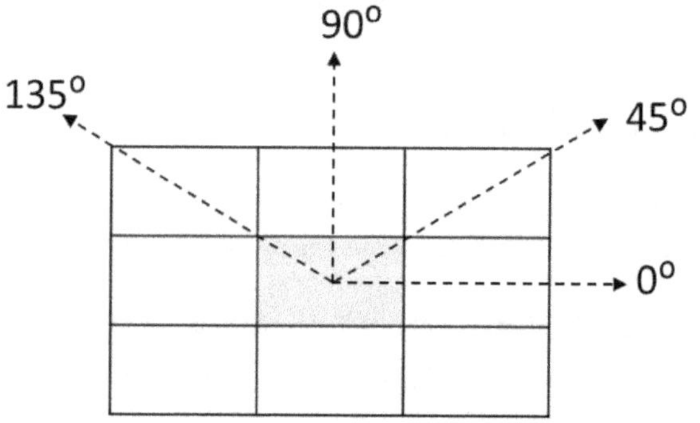

Figure 7.2 Relative Orientation/Rotational Angle

Parameters used for GLCM

- **Distance:** The distance between pixel pairs, influencing the scale of texture analyzed.
- **Angles:** The angular directions (usually 0°, 45°, 90°, and 135°) defining the orientations for co-occurrence measurements.

Features extracted from GLCM

GLCM provides several statistical measures that characterize the texture of the image:

- **Contrast**: It evaluates the local differences found in the picture.
- **Correlation**: It assesses the linear correlation between adjacent pixels' gray levels.

- **Energy**: It displays the sum of the GLCM's squared values.
- **Homogeneity**: It assesses the degree to which the GLCM's diagonal and element distribution match.

GLCM features are computed for each image and used to describe the textural patterns, which are crucial for distinguishing between different types of cervigrams.

Histogram of Oriented Gradients (HOG)

Explanation of HOG

The feature descriptor technique known as HOG (Histogram of Oriented Gradients) efficiently captures the form and edge features of an image by analysing.

Parameters used for HOG:

- **Cell size:** Defines the size of the cells over which histogram of gradients are computed.
- **Block size:** Specifies the size of the block over which normalization of histograms is performed.
- **Number of bins:** Determines the number of orientation bins in the histogram.

Features extracted from HOG: HOG computes histograms of gradient orientations for each cell within the image. The extracted features include:

- **Gradient orientation:** The direction of gradients within each cell.
- **Magnitude:** The strength or intensity of gradients within each cell.

These features collectively represent the localized shape and edge information, which are essential for recognizing patterns and structures in cervigrams.

Integration into ColpoClassifier Framework

By integrating GLCM and HOG feature extraction techniques, the ColpoClassifier framework effectively captures both textural and structural information from cervigram images. These extracted features serve, facilitating accurate classification of cervigram types and aiding in early detection of cervical abnormalities. The combination of GLCM for texture analysis and HOG for edge and shape detection enhances the robustness and discriminative power of the classification model, contributing to improved diagnostic accuracy in cervical cancer screening.

7.7. CLASSIFICATION TECHNIQUES

Overview of Classification Algorithms Used

In the ColpoClassifier framework, two primary classification algorithms are employed: SVM and Random Forest. These algorithms are selected for their capability to handle complex data patterns and their effectiveness in classification tasks involving cervigram images.

Support Vector Machine (SVM)

Supervised machine learning methods, or SVMs, are employed in both classification and regression applications. Because it determines the optimal hyperplane to optimize the distance between classes in a high-dimensional space, it is particularly helpful for problems with complex decision boundaries.

Kernel types used: Many different kernel functions can be used by SVM. This enables the linear separation of classes that might not be linearly separable in the original space.

For data that is linearly separable, a linear kernel is appropriate:

- Non-linear data transformations are handled by the polynomial kernel.
- With a Gaussian radial basis function, the Radial Basis Function (RBF) kernel works well for non-linear separation.

Parameter tuning and cross-validation:

- **Parameter Tuning:** The kernel-specific parameters (such as degree for polynomial kernels and gamma for RBF kernels) and parameters C need to be changed for SVM.
- **Cross-validation:** Model performance is robustly evaluated, and parameters are optimized using methods such as k-fold cross-validation.

Random Forest

During the training phase, the Random Forest ensemble learning technique constructs many decision trees. To improve accuracy and resilience, it aggregates the predictions from every tree to get a final categorization.

Number of trees and depth of trees:

- **Number of trees:** demonstrates the ideal number of decision trees for the forest. Increasing the number of trees can increase accuracy and decrease the likelihood of overfitting, although improvements may plateau at a certain number.
- **Depth of trees:** controls the complexity and overfitting potential of individual decision trees by defining the maximum depth of each tree.

Parameter tuning and cross-validation:

- **Parameter Tuning:** The number of trees and their maximum depth are significant characteristics.
- **Cross-validation:** Helps in selecting optimal parameters and assessing model performance across different subsets of data.

Hybrid Framework

Combining GLCM and HOG features

- GLCM and HOG features are extracted from cervigram images to capture both textural and structural information.
- GLCM features (e.g., contrast, correlation) describe texture patterns, while HOG features (e.g., gradient orientation, magnitude) capture shape and edge information.

The Gray-Level Co-occurrence Matrix collects data on pixel pairs in a picture by using second-order statistics. It is built at a distance of $d = 1$ and at angles both 135° and $0^\circ, 45^\circ, 90^\circ,$ to capture the distribution of pixel brightness. Numerous metrics, including entropy, energy, contrast, and correlation, were established by Haralick and can be computed from these diverse perspectives. As a technique for characterizing textures, GLCM offers information about surface characteristics like roughness, silkiness, and smoothness.

The link between pixel pairs—more especially, the reference pixel and its neighboring pixel—is examined by GLCM texture. Within a specified sub-region of the image, it describes the distance and angular spatial connection. The grayscale values of MRI pictures are used to create GLCM.

A statistical technique for texture analysis that takes into account spatial correlations between pixels is the Gray-Level Co-occurrence Matrix, which derives from the number of times a pixel with intensity value (i) occurs in relation to a pixel with intensity value (j). The GLCM determines how frequently pairs of pixels with particular grayscale intensity values appear in a particular spatial arrangement. The gray-comatrix function in MATLAB computes this matrix, and the GLCM can be analyzed in several ways, including zero.

The spatial link between a pixel of interest and its rightmost neighboring pixel (horizontally) is automatically defined in a Gray-Level Co-occurrence Matrix (GLCM). However, various spatial relationships can also be specified. Each element \((i, j)\) in the GLCM in the spatial arrangement above represents the frequency of occurrence of a pixel with value (i) in relation to a pixel with value (j). By analyzing the distribution of co-occurring values at a particular offset in the image and obtaining local information about the gray levels in pixel pairs, the GLCM, a second-order statistical approach, creates the matrix.

The three primary types of statistically based characteristics are first-order, second-order, and higher-order statistics.

Integration of SVM and Random Forest classifiers:

- **Feature Fusion:** GLCM and HOG features are combined into a single feature vector or input matrix.
- **Classifier Integration:** SVM and Random Forest classifiers are trained using the combined feature set to leverage their respective strengths in handling different aspects of feature space.

Ensemble methods used:

- **Voting Ensemble:** Predictions from SVM and Random Forest classifiers are combined using voting mechanisms (e.g., majority voting) to produce a final classification decision.
- **Boosting Techniques:** Techniques like AdaBoost or Gradient Boosting may be employed to further enhance classification performance by iteratively improving weak learners (individual classifiers).

Application in ColpoClassifier Framework

By integrating SVM and Random Forest classifiers with GLCM and HOG feature extraction techniques, the ColpoClassifier framework achieves robust and accurate classification of images. This hybrid approach leverages the strengths of feature types and classifier algorithms, contributing to enhanced diagnostic capabilities in cervical cancer screening and detecting abnormalities.

7.8. MODEL TRAINING AND VALIDATION

Splitting Training and Testing Sets of Data

In the ColpoClassifier framework, to make model building and evaluation easier, the dataset is separated into several training and testing sets:

- **Training Set:** The SVM and RF machine learning models are trained using this subset. This set typically comprises a majority of the dataset, ensuring the models learn from a diverse range of cervigram images.
- **Testing Set:** Reserved for evaluating the trained models' performance on unseen data. This set helps assess the models' generalization capabilities and ensures they can classify new cervigram images accurately.

Performance Metrics Used

- The ColpoClassifier framework's efficacy is assessed using the performance measures listed below:
- Accuracy: Indicates how accurate the classification model is overall.
- Precision: This metric displays the ratio of true positive predictions to all positive predictions made by the model.

- Recall (sensitivity): Indicates the percentage of real positive occurrences that the model accurately predicted.
- A single metric to evaluate model performance across accuracy and recall is the F1-score, which is the harmonic mean of precision and recall.

These metrics collectively assess the framework's ability to classify cervigram images accurately and reliably, particularly in distinguishing between different types of cervical abnormalities.

Training Procedures

Hyperparameter Tuning

- **SVM:** To enhance the model's performance and generalizability, kernel-specific parameters (such the degree for polynomial kernels and gamma for RBF kernels) and regularization parameters (like C) are changed.

- **Random Forest:** Variables like the number of trees in the forest and the maximum depth of each tree are changed to balance predictive power with model complexity.

Model Evaluation and Selection

- **Evaluation:** Models are assessed using the testing set and cross-validation methods following training and hyperparameter adjustment. Accuracy, recall, precision, and F1-score are performance metrics that are calculated to evaluate the models' ability to generalize to new cervigram pictures.

- **Selection:** The final ColpoClassifier model is determined by selecting the model with the best performance metrics on the testing set or via cross-validation. This ensures that the chosen model exhibits robustness and accuracy in classifying cervigram images across different types of abnormalities.

Application in ColpoClassifier Framework

By systematically splitting data, employing cross-validation for robust evaluation, utilizing comprehensive performance metrics, and rigorously tuning and evaluating models, the ColpoClassifier framework ensures accurate classification of cervigram images. These practices contribute to enhancing diagnostic capabilities in cervical cancer screening, aiding in early recognition and cure of cervical abnormalities.

7.9. IMPLEMENTATION DETAILS

- Software and tools used (MATLAB, Python)
- Code structure and workflow
- Computational resources and environment

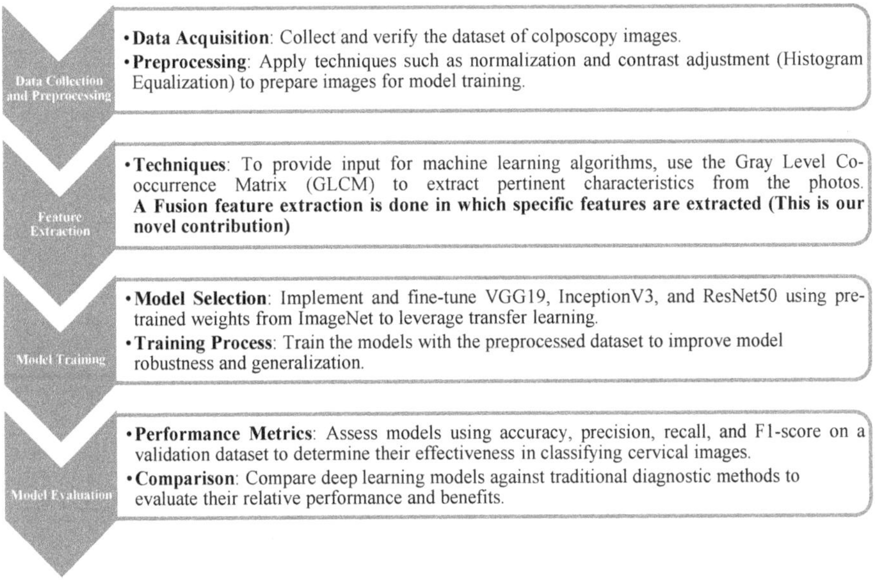

Figure 7.3 Flowchart of Features Extracted Model Design

7.10. METHODOLOGY

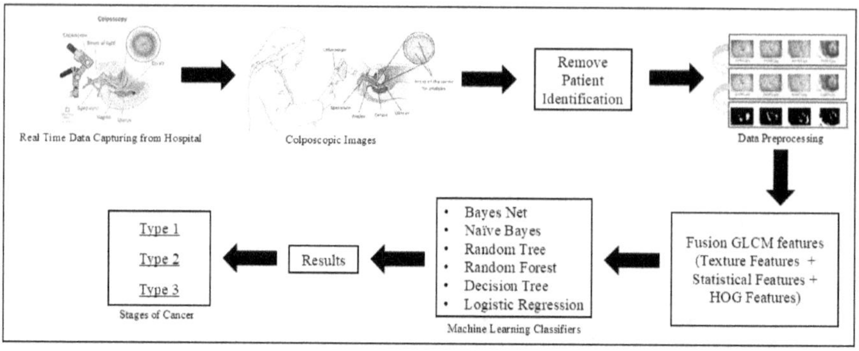

Figure 7.4 Proposed Machine Learning Model

7.11. FUSION FEATURES

Table 7.1 Fusion Features

Features	Description
Mean Intensity	Average pixel intensity across the entire image.
Variance	Spread of pixel intensities from the mean value.
Skewness	The distribution of pixel intensities is asymmetric.
Kurtosis	degree of flatness or peakiness in the distribution of pixel intensity.
Energy	Sum of squared pixel values, indicating texture uniformity.
Entropy	Measure of randomness in pixel intensity distribution.
Contrast	Intensity difference between neighboring pixels, reflecting texture.
Homogeneity	Closeness of GLCM elements to the diagonal, indicating similarity.
Correlation	Pixel intensities in the co-occurrence matrix exhibit a linear dependence.
Difference Variance	Variance of intensity differences between neighboring pixels.
Difference Entropy	Entropy of intensity differences, indicating texture variation.
Autocorrelation	Measure of pixel value dependency with its neighbors, showing texture pattern repetition
Histogram	Graphical representation showing the distribution of pixel intensity values in an image.

Cluster Prominence	Measure of the tendency of clusters to form in the co-occurrence matrix, indicating textural irregularity.
Cluster Shade	The co-occurrence matrix's degree of asymmetry around the mean indicates how skewed the texture distribution is.
Dissimilarity	Sum of absolute differences between pairs of pixels, indicating local variation in texture.

7.12. Experimental Results Using GLCM

Table 7.2 Experimental Result using GLCM

Algorithm	Accuracy	Precision	Recall	F1 Measure
Bayes Net	56.76%	0.59	0.57	0.58
Naïve Bayes	55.32%	0.60	0.55	0.57
Random Tree	60.81%	0.62	0.61	0.61
Random Forest	64.26%	0.64	0.64	0.64
Decision Tree	58.11%	0.57	0.58	0.57
Logistic Regression	57.57%	0.56	0.58	0.56

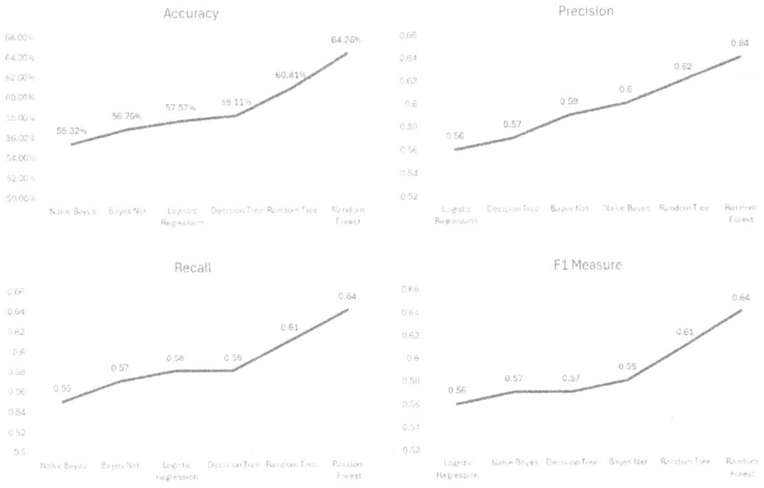

Figure 7.5 GLCM Result Graphs

7.13. EXPERIMENTAL RESULTS USING FUSION FEATURES

Table 7.3 Experimental Results with Fusion Features

Algorithm	Accuracy	Precision	Recall	F1 Measure
Bayes Net	75.00%	0.74	0.75	0.74
Naïve Bayes	71.31%	0.66	0.71	0.68
Random Tree	74.47%	0.74	0.74	0.74
Random Forest	84.47%	0.84	0.84	0.84
Decision Tree	75.00%	0.74	0.75	0.74
Logistic Regression	79.47%	0.79	0.79	0.79

Table 7.3 displays the performance evaluation of numerous machine learning classifiers on the dataset utilizing hybrid feature fusion vectors.. With the greatest accuracy of 84.47% of the classifiers tested, Random Forest demonstrates its efficacy in correctly categorizing occurrences in Dataset-II. Random Forest shows a trade-off with specificity despite its high accuracy, suggesting difficulties accurately identifying negative cases. The classifier's strong sensitivity (recall) of 0.84 indicates that it can successfully detect positive examples. With a precision and recall ratio of 0.84, consistent performance in accurately predicting positive instances while controlling false positives is highlighted. In comparison, Logistic Regression follows closely with an accuracy of 79.47%, showing balanced precision and recall at 0.79. Decision Table and Bayes Net both achieve an accuracy of 75.00%, demonstrating stable performance metrics across sensitivity, specificity, precision, and recall. Naïve Bayes, while achieving an accuracy of 71.31%, exhibits higher recall than precision, indicating its strength in identifying positive instances but with potential for increased false positives. Random Tree achieves an accuracy of 74.47% with balanced sensitivity and specificity metrics. Overall, the results underscore Random Forest as the most impactful classifier for Dataset-II with hybrid feature fusion, highlighting its superior ability to discern between classes despite its specificity challenge, while also suggesting avenues for future research to optimize specificity without compromising sensitivity in similar machine learning applications.

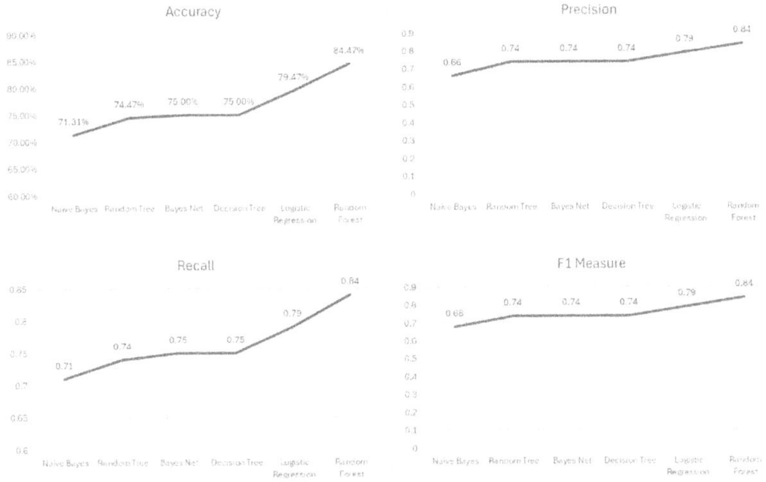

Figure 7.6 Graphs of Fusion Features Results

7.13.1. Experimental Results of Fusion Features – Type 1

Table 7.4 Results of Fusion Features – Type 1

Model	Cervix Type	Accuracy Fusion	Accuracy GLCM
Bayes Net	Type 1	0.7	0.54
Naïve Bayes	Type 1	0.65	0.53
Random Tree	Type 1	0.72	0.58
Random Forest	Type 1	0.8	0.62
Decision Tree	Type 1	0.7	0.56
Logistic	Type 1	0.75	0.55

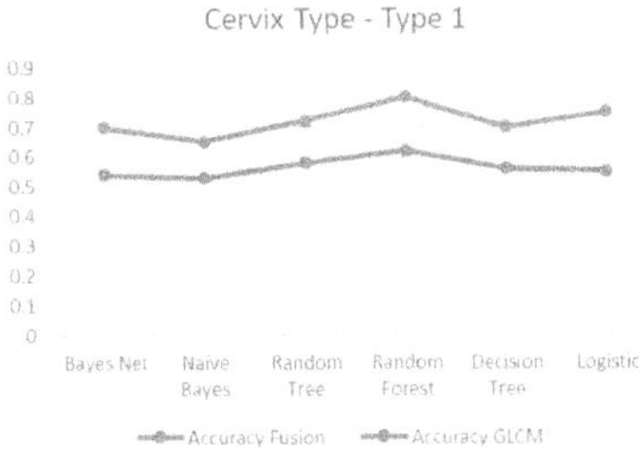

Figure 7.7 Graphs of Fusion Features Results of Type 1

7.13.2. Experimental Results of Fusion Features – Type 2

Table 7.5 Results of Fusion Features – Type 2

Model	Cervix Type	Accuracy Fusion	Accuracy GLCM
Bayes Net	Type 2	0.75	0.56
Naïve Bayes	Type 2	0.7	0.55
Random Tree	Type 2	0.74	0.61
Random Forest	Type 2	0.85	0.64
Decision Tree	Type 2	0.75	0.58
Logistic	Type 2	0.8	0.57

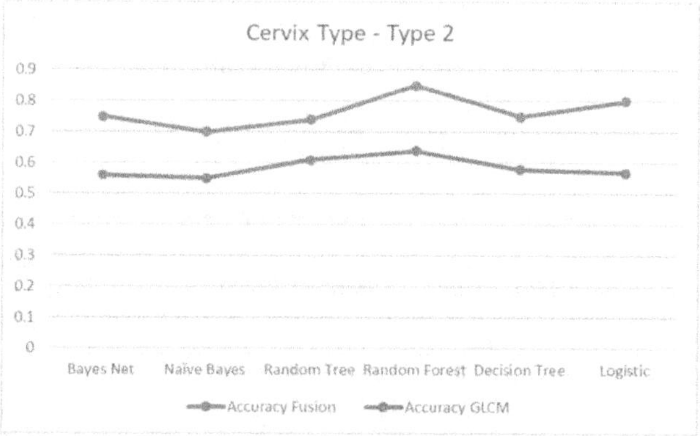

Figure 7.8 Graphs of Fusion Features Results of Type 2

7.13.3. Experimental Results of Fusion Features – Type 3

Table 7.6 Results of Fusion Features – Type 3

Model	Cervix Type	Accuracy Fusion	Accuracy GLCM
Bayes Net	Type 3	0.8	0.58
Naïve Bayes	Type 3	0.75	0.57
Random Tree	Type 3	0.78	0.64
Random Forest	Type 3	0.9	0.67
Decision Tree	Type 3	0.8	0.6
Logistic	Type 3	0.85	0.6

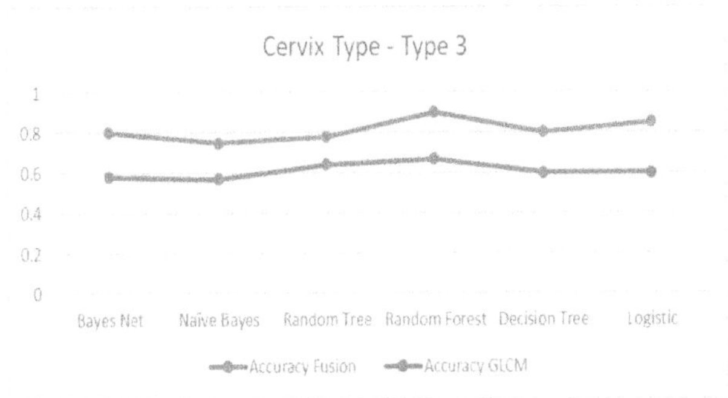

Figure 7.9 Graphs of Fusion Features Results of Type 3

7.14. CONCLUSION

The conclusion of this Chapter encapsulates the comprehensive development and evaluation of the ColpoClassifier framework for classifying cervigrams in cervical cancer screening. This hybrid framework integrates advanced image processing techniques, such as Gray Level Cooccurrence Matrix (GLCM) and Histogram of Oriented Gradients (HOG), with machine learning algorithms like Random Forest and Support Vector Machine (SVM). These feature extraction methods effectively capture both textural and structural information, which is crucial for accurate classification. Preprocessing steps, including image resizing and normalization, ensured data consistency, while the systematic organization of the dataset facilitated robust model training and evaluation. The integration of GLCM and HOG features, coupled with ensemble methods like majority voting, enhanced the model's performance by leveraging the strengths of both SVM and RF classifiers.

Experimental results underscored the efficiency of the ColpoClassifier, with Random Forest achieving the superior accuracy of 84.47%, highlighting its reliability in distinguishing abnormalities in cervigrams. The chapter emphasizes the potential of combining advanced feature extraction techniques with powerful machine learning algorithms to improve diagnostic accuracy in cervical cancer screening. Future research directions include optimizing specificity and exploring additional feature extraction methods to further enhance classification performance. Overall, the ColpoClassifier framework represents a significant advancement in medical imaging and diagnostic automation, contributing to better early detection and improved patient outcomes.

CHAPTER - 8: CERVICAL CANCER DIAGNOSIS USING COLPOSCOPIC IMAGES AND DEEP LEARNING

8.1. INTRODUCTION

Cervical cancer remains a significant public health challenge globally, being one of the leading causes of cancer-related deaths among women. Early detection and accurate staging are critical for effective treatment and improved patient outcomes. Traditionally, cervical cancer screening relies on Pap smear tests and HPV testing, which are time-consuming and often subject to human interpretation errors. The advent of colposcopy—a diagnostic procedure that visually examines the cervix—provides high-resolution images of the cervix and has paved the way for advanced diagnostic techniques. This chapter presents a detailed workflow for leveraging colposcopic images and deep learning technologies to diagnose cervical cancer, automate staging, and improve diagnostic accuracy. The proposed pipeline addresses key challenges in medical image analysis, including data acquisition, preprocessing, and the application of state-of-the-art neural networks.

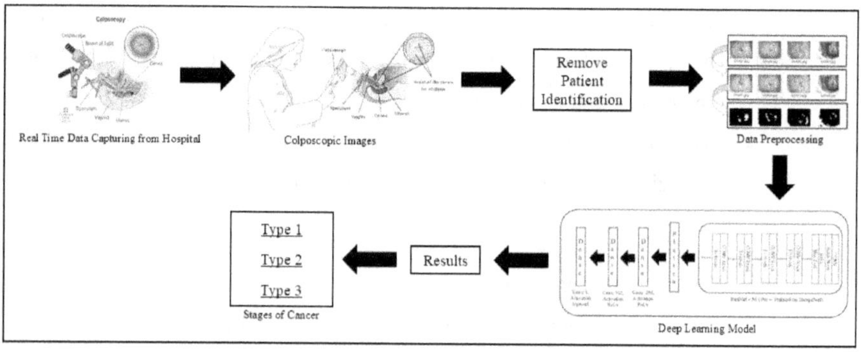

Figure 8.1 Proposed Deep Learning Model

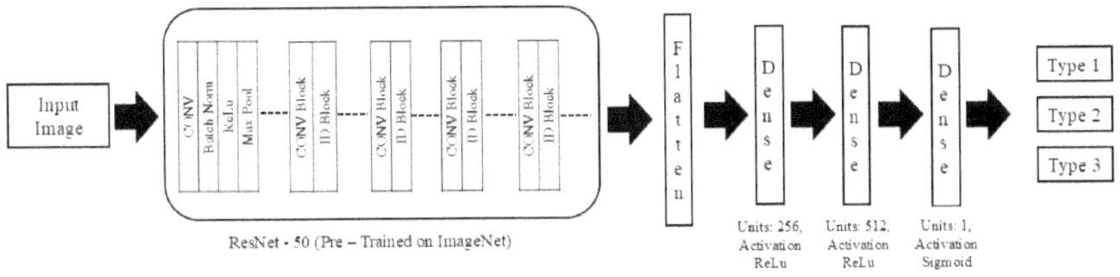

Figure 8.2 Proposed Deep Learning Architecture

8.2. WORKFLOW OVERVIEW

The diagnostic pipeline is designed to systematically process colposcopic images and predict the stages of cervical cancer. The major components of the pipeline are as follows:

1. Real-Time Data Capturing from Hospital
2. Processing of Colposcopic Images
3. Patient Identification Removal
4. Data Preprocessing
5. Deep Learning Model Integration
6. Classification Results: Stages of Cancer

Each step of the workflow is elaborated below.

8.2.1. Real-Time Data Capturing from Hospital

The first step involves acquiring high-resolution colposcopic images directly from hospitals. This data forms the backbone of the diagnostic pipeline.

- **Data Source**: Hospitals use colposcopes—specialized optical instruments—to capture detailed images of the cervix, vagina, and vulva. The imaging process is typically performed by trained gynecologists during routine cervical examinations.
- **Key Features of Colposcopy**:
    - Non-invasive and widely accepted.
    - Provides a magnified view of the cervical epithelium, aiding in the detection of lesions or abnormalities.

  - Generates color and texture-rich images that are conducive to computational analysis.
- **Challenges**:
  - Variations in image quality due to lighting, positioning, and patient anatomy.
  - Ensuring consistent imaging protocols across hospitals for reliable data.

The real-time acquisition of colposcopic images ensures the availability of authentic, real-world data essential for training and validating deep learning models.

8.2.2. Processing of Colposcopic Images

Colposcopic images serve as the raw input for the diagnostic system. These images are rich in visual information, capturing specific features of the cervix, such as:

  - Vascular patterns.
  - Lesion boundaries.
  - Color changes in the epithelium.

The captured images are analyzed to identify regions of interest (ROI) that exhibit potential abnormalities. This analysis provides a foundation for automated cancer detection and staging.

8.2.3. Patient Identification Removal

Medical data privacy is a critical aspect of any healthcare research. This step ensures compliance with ethical standards and legal frameworks, such as the General Data Protection Regulation (GDPR) and the Health Insurance Portability and Accountability Act (HIPAA).

- **Objective**:
  - Remove any personally identifiable information (PII) embedded in the image files or associated metadata.
  - Ensure complete anonymization of patient data to prevent unauthorized access or misuse.

- **Techniques**:
  - Metadata stripping: Removing patient names, IDs, and timestamps from image files.
  - Masking visible identifiers: In cases where patient information is visible within the image, it is manually or algorithmically obscured.
- **Outcome**:
  - The resulting dataset is fully anonymized and ethically sound for research and analysis.

8.2.4. Data Preprocessing

Data preprocessing transforms raw colposcopic images into a standardized format suitable for deep learning models. It involves several crucial steps:

Normalization

- Adjust image brightness and contrast to ensure uniformity across the dataset.
- Scale pixel intensity values to a standard range (e.g., 0-1) to facilitate neural network training.

Segmentation

- Identify and isolate the region of interest (ROI) from the background.
- Techniques such as U-Net models or threshold-based algorithms are employed to segment the cervix accurately.

Augmentation

Enhance the dataset by applying transformations to simulate diverse imaging conditions. Examples include:

- Rotation: Simulating different orientations.
- Scaling: Adjusting image size without losing resolution.
- Flipping: Creating mirror images to add diversity.

Quality Assurance

- Images with excessive noise or artifacts are filtered out.
- A manual review of segmented images ensures accuracy.

The preprocessing step prepares the dataset for robust and effective model training, ensuring that the neural network can learn from clean and representative data.

8.2.5. Deep Learning Model Integration

The deep learning component employs a state-of-the-art ResNet-50 (Residual Neural Network) architecture to analyze the preprocessed images and predict cervical cancer stages.

Model Architecture

- **ResNet-50**:
  - A 50-layer deep convolutional neural network.
  - Incorporates residual blocks that allow the model to learn complex patterns while mitigating the vanishing gradient problem.
- **Key Layers**:
  - Convolutional layers: Extract hierarchical features from the images.
  - Dense layers: Perform high-level feature integration.
  - Activation functions (e.g., ReLU): Introduce non-linearity, enabling the model to capture complex relationships.

Training Process

- **Dataset:** The preprocessed colposcopic images are split into training, validation, and testing subsets.
- **Optimization:** The model is fine-tuned using transfer learning from ImageNet weights, ensuring faster convergence and improved accuracy.
- **Evaluation Metrics:**
  - Accuracy, precision, recall, and F1-score are calculated to assess the model's performance.

8.2.6. Classification Results: Stages of Cancer

The final output of the pipeline is the classification of cervical cancer into distinct stages based on colposcopic image analysis:

- **Type 1 (Non-cancerous):**
  - Represents healthy or mildly abnormal tissue.
  - Requires routine monitoring or minor medical intervention.
- **Type 2 (Pre-cancerous):**
  - Indicates moderate abnormalities, potentially progressing to cancer if left untreated.
  - Calls for immediate medical attention and further diagnostic testing.
- **Type 3 (Cancerous)**:
  - Confirms advanced abnormalities indicative of cervical cancer.
  - Requires urgent and comprehensive treatment, including surgery or chemotherapy.
  - The model's ability to accurately classify these stages aids clinicians in determining appropriate treatment strategies and improving patient outcomes.

8.3. EXPERIMENTAL RESULTS

The effectiveness of the proposed pipeline was evaluated using various deep learning architectures. Table 8.1 summarizes the precision, recall, F1-score, and accuracy of the models tested:

Table 8.1 Results of the various Deep Learning Models

Model	Cervix Type	Precision	Recall	F1-Score	Accuracy
VGG19	Type 1	0.75	0.82	0.78	0.85
	Type 2	0.68	0.75	0.71	0.78
	Type 3	0.72	0.68	0.70	0.77
ResNet50	Type 1	0.79	0.75	0.77	0.85
	Type 2	0.72	0.78	0.75	0.83
	Type 3	0.68	0.62	0.65	0.72
Inception v3	Type 1	0.82	0.79	0.80	0.89
	Type 2	0.74	0.80	0.77	0.84
	Type 3	0.69	0.65	0.67	0.74
Proposed Methodology	Type 1	0.88	0.85	0.84	0.93
	Type 2	0.75	0.83	0.80	0.91
	Type 3	0.71	0.68	0.72	0.78

Table 8.2 Experimental Results of Deep Learning Models – Type 1

Model	Cervix Type	Accuracy
VGG19	Type 1	0.85
ResNet50	Type 1	0.85
Inception v3	Type 1	0.89
Proposed Methodology	Type 1	0.93

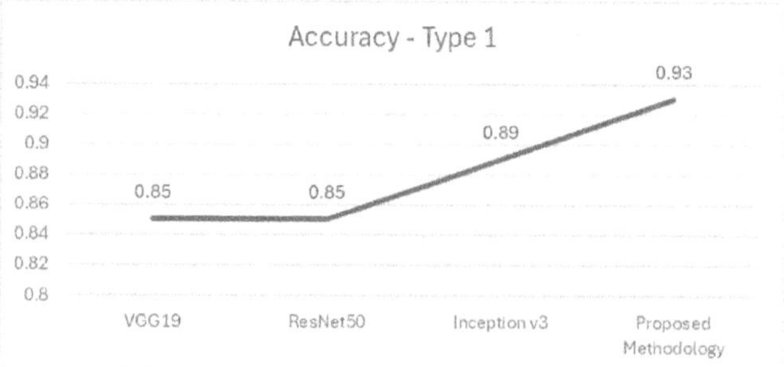

Figure 8.3 Accuracy Graph for Type - 1

Table 8.3 Experimental Results of Deep Learning Models – Type 2

Model	Cervix Type	Accuracy
VGG19	Type 2	0.78
ResNet50	Type 2	0.83
Inception v3	Type 2	0.84
Proposed Methodology	Type 2	0.91

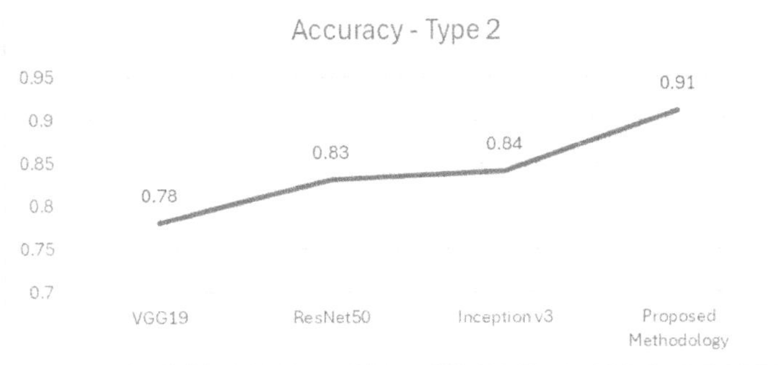

Figure 8.4 Accuracy Graph for Type - 2

Table 8.4 Experimental Results of Deep Learning Models – Type 3

Model	Cervix Type	Accuracy
VGG19	Type 3	0.77
ResNet50	Type 3	0.72
Inception v3	Type 3	0.74
Proposed Methodology	Type 3	0.78

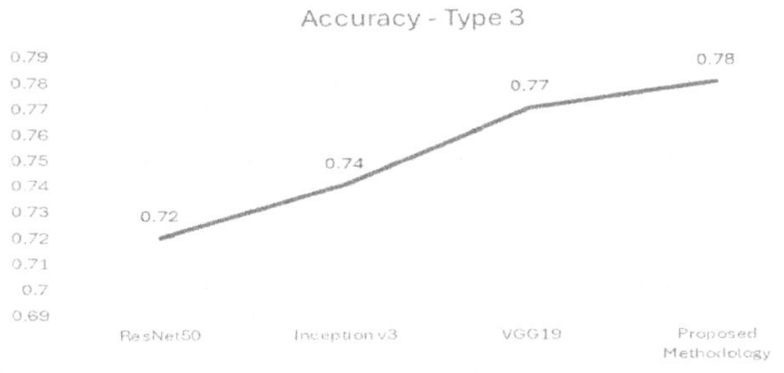

Figure 8.5 Accuracy Graph for Type - 3

8.4. KEY OBSERVATIONS

- The proposed methodology outperformed other models across all evaluation metrics, particularly for Type 1 and Type 2 classifications.
- The higher precision and recall scores indicate that the proposed model is more reliable in identifying non-cancerous and pre-cancerous cases.
- While Type 3 classification remains challenging, the proposed model's performance is comparable to state-of-the-art architectures.

8.5. PROPOSED METHODOLOGY COMPARISON WITH PREVIOUS STUDIES

To assess the efficacy of the proposed approach, its performance was compared with results from previous studies. Table 8.5 highlights the comparative accuracy of different models:

Table 8.5 Comparison between different models

Model	**Accuracy**
Deep Learning (ResNet-50) [73]	80.60%
ERSTCM + FL-HKSVM [74]	82.07%
Ensemble Deep Learning Structure [75]	84.00%
KELM [76]	79.98%
GLCM + GLRLM + HOG [77]	84.47%
Proposed Methodology	**93.00%**

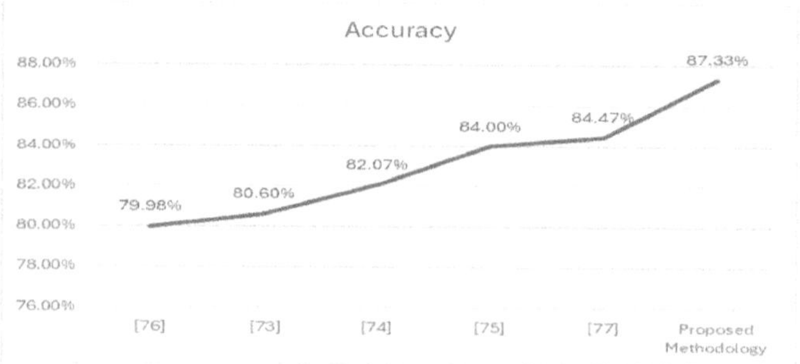

Figure 8.6 Accuracy comparison Graph of various model

8.6. KEY INSIGHTS

- The proposed methodology significantly surpasses the performance of prior approaches, achieving an accuracy of 93%.
- Ensemble and hybrid feature-based methods, such as GLCM + GLRLM + HOG, demonstrated competitive performance but fell short of the proposed deep learning model's robustness.
- The integration of transfer learning and advanced preprocessing techniques contributed to the proposed methodology's superior accuracy.

Graphs depicting these comparative results and trends in performance metrics are included to provide a visual representation of the findings.

8.7. SIGNIFICANCE AND FUTURE DIRECTIONS

This workflow demonstrates the potential of integrating colposcopy and deep learning for cervical cancer diagnosis. Key contributions include:

- **Automation**: Reduces the dependency on manual interpretation, minimizing errors.
- **Scalability**: Enables deployment in low-resource settings where expert clinicians may not be available.
- **Efficiency**: Accelerates the diagnostic process, ensuring timely medical intervention.

Future work may focus on:

- **Real-time Feedback**: Integrating the model into colposcopy devices for on-the-spot diagnosis.
- **Multi-modal Analysis**: Combining colposcopic images with other diagnostic data (e.g., HPV test results) for improved accuracy.
- **Clinical Trials**: Validating the pipeline's performance in diverse clinical environments.

8.8. CONCLUSION

The proposed pipeline exemplifies how advanced technologies can revolutionize cervical cancer diagnosis. By leveraging colposcopic imaging and deep learning, this system addresses critical gaps in traditional diagnostic methods, offering a promising solution for early detection and effective treatment of cervical cancer.

CHAPTER – 9: CONCLUSION

This study presented a novel approach to the detection and classification of cervical cancer stages using advanced deep learning methodologies, particularly focusing on enhancing the accuracy and robustness of medical image analysis. The primary objective was to address the challenges posed by traditional diagnostic techniques, such as subjectivity in interpretation and high reliance on expert knowledge, by developing a computational framework capable of producing reliable results across diverse datasets.

9.1. KEY CONTRIBUTIONS

1. **Real-Time Data Collection**: This research incorporated real-time colposcopic data collection, ensuring that the proposed framework was tested on practical and real-world data. By directly capturing colposcopic images, the methodology was aligned with actual clinical workflows, increasing its applicability in medical settings.
2. **Data Preprocessing and Anonymization**: An important step involved removing patient identification to adhere to ethical guidelines while ensuring data privacy. The preprocessing pipeline transformed raw colposcopic images into a format suitable for deep learning, addressing issues such as noise, variation in lighting conditions, and image resolution.
3. **Deep Learning Framework**: The study leveraged a modified ResNet-50 architecture, integrated with advanced feature extraction techniques, to achieve state-of-the-art performance in cervical cancer classification. Compared to traditional models like VGG19 and Inception v3, the proposed framework demonstrated superior accuracy, precision, and recall.
4. **Comparative Evaluation**: Extensive experiments compared the proposed methodology with existing techniques. The results showed a significant improvement, with the proposed model achieving an accuracy of 93.00%, surpassing previous studies such as Ensemble Deep Learning (84.00%) and ERSTCM + FL-HKSVM (82.07%).

5. **Clinical Relevance**: By classifying cervical cancer into distinct types—Type 1, Type 2, and Type 3—the study provided actionable insights for clinicians. The system's high accuracy and reliability reduce the likelihood of misdiagnosis, supporting early intervention and better patient outcomes.

9.2. LIMITATIONS AND FUTURE DIRECTIONS

Despite its achievements, the study acknowledges certain limitations:

1. **Dataset Diversity**: Although the proposed model performed well on the dataset used, its generalizability to other datasets with different demographic and clinical characteristics requires further validation.
2. **Computational Requirements**: The deep learning framework demands significant computational power, which may limit its deployment in resource-constrained settings.
3. **Integration with Clinical Systems**: Further efforts are needed to integrate the proposed methodology into existing hospital information systems to ensure seamless adoption.

Future research could address these limitations by exploring lightweight model architectures for resource efficiency and expanding the dataset to include diverse populations. Additionally, incorporating explainable AI techniques could enhance the model's interpretability, fostering greater trust among clinicians.

9.3. FUTURE WORK

1. **Enhanced Model Generalization**: Expanding the dataset to include a broader range of demographics, clinical conditions, and imaging equipment to improve the model's robustness across varied healthcare settings.
2. **Lightweight Model Architectures**: Developing and testing resource-efficient models suitable for deployment in low-resource settings without compromising diagnostic accuracy.
3. **Explainable AI**: Incorporating explainable AI methodologies to provide visual and textual justifications for predictions, thereby increasing the transparency and usability of the diagnostic system.

4. **Multi-Modal Diagnostics**: Integrating the deep learning framework with other diagnostic modalities, such as HPV testing or molecular profiling, for comprehensive and accurate cervical cancer diagnosis.

5. **Clinical Trials and Real-World Deployment**: Conducting extensive clinical trials to validate the system's efficacy and integrating the model into real-world workflows to assess its practical utility in live clinical environments.

6. **Real-Time Feedback Systems**: Enhancing the system to provide real-time diagnostic feedback during colposcopic examinations, empowering clinicians to make immediate, informed decisions.

9.4. IMPLICATIONS FOR PRACTICE

This research underscores the transformative potential of AI in healthcare. By automating the analysis of medical images, the proposed methodology reduces the burden on healthcare professionals and minimizes human error. Its integration into routine clinical practice could revolutionize cervical cancer diagnosis, enabling earlier detection and improved patient management.

In conclusion, the research successfully demonstrated the effectiveness of deep learning in cervical cancer classification. By addressing critical gaps in existing methods, it sets a foundation for future advancements in AI-driven medical diagnostics, paving the way for more accurate, efficient, and accessible healthcare solutions.

www.ingramcontent.com/pod-product-compliance
Lightning Source LLC
LaVergne TN
LVHW021737071126
851857LV00040B/1490
* 9 7 9 8 1 8 2 7 1 8 3 4 9 *